W9-AUW-580

Voices of Breast Cancer

The Healing Companion:
Stories for Courage,
Comfort and Strength

Other Books by the Healing Project

Voices of Alzheimer's

Voices of Lung Cancer

Voices of Breast Cancer

The Healing Companion: Stories for Courage, Comfort and Strength

Edited by

The Healing Project

www.thehealingproject.org

"Voices Of" Series Book No. 3

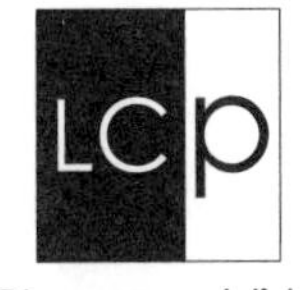

LaChance publishing

LACHANCE PUBLISHING • NEW YORK
www.lachancepublishing.com

Copyright © 2007 by LaChance Publishing LLC

ISBN 978-1-934184-00-4

All rights reserved. Printed in the United States of America.

No portion of this book may be reproduced—mechanically, electronically, or by any other means, including photocopying—without the express written permission of the publisher.

Library of Congress Control Number: 2007928038

Publisher: LaChance Publishing LLC
120 Bond Street
Brooklyn, NY 11201
www.lachancepublishing.com

Distributor: Independent Publishers Group
814 North Franklin Street
Chicago, IL 60610
www.ipgbook.com

Victor Starsia
Managing Editor

Richard Day Gore
Editor

All things have a beginning and sometimes the journey from beginning to end is not always clear and straightforward. While work on *Voices Of* began just two years ago, the seeds were planted long ago by beloved sources. This book is dedicated to Jennie, Larry and Denise, who in the face of all things good and bad gave courage and support in excess. And especially to Richard, who taught us by the way he lived his life that anything is possible given enough time, hard work and love.

Contents

Part I: FINDING OUT

Part II: BREAKING THE NEWS

Part III: I'VE CHANGED

Part IV: HOW DO I DEAL WITH THIS?

Part V: I AM TAKING CHARGE

Part VI: I AM A SURVIVOR

Foreword
Living Beyond Breast Cancer
Jean A. Sachs, MSS, MLSP

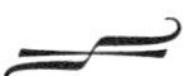

Much has changed in our approach to breast cancer in the fifteen years since the founding of Living Beyond Breast Cancer. During this tumultuous period, women diagnosed with the disease and their families, friends and supporters established and grew effective non-profit organizations focused on raising public awareness, garnering funds for research, ensuring access to quality medical care and providing education and support for those affected by the disease. They demanded, and received, an increase in government funding for breast cancer research and broke through the ranks of the established scientific community to get women with breast cancer a "seat at the table" where research decisions are made. National Breast Cancer Awareness Month has helped to further raise awareness: each October more newspapers, magazines, store fronts and products are covered with pink ribbons, more women walk hundreds of miles to raise money for research and more companies donate millions of dollars to our cause.

Increased funding has resulted in research developments that have changed the way we treat and manage breast cancer. Doctors perform more lumpectomies, sparing some women the loss of their breast. Biotechnology companies have developed tests that help doctors predict which cancers will better respond to chemotherapy. The discovery of aromatase inhibitors and targeted therapies like trastuzumab (Herceptin®) and lapatinib (Tykerb®) have revolutionized the way we think about breast cancer. Today we expect, and demand, more focused treatments that allow women to get the best result while maintaining an excellent quality of life.

Despite all our achievements, however, breast cancer remains a serious health concern. It continues to top the list of women's cancers. The American Cancer Society estimates that 200,000 women and 1,700 men will be diagnosed with breast cancer in 2007. And this year alone, more than 40,000 will die of advanced, or metastatic, disease.

As an advocate, I refuse to be satisfied until we eradicate all forms of breast cancer. But I also know my job is much more than fighting for an end to disease. It is about helping the women who face this disease now, and statistics and pink ribbons don't tell their story. Statistics don't show how a diagnosis can rock a family to its core, or change the course of a relationship, or shake the foundations of a friendship. Among the masses of pink ribbons are the individual stories, often forgotten, of women and families coping with this life-threatening and often life-changing disease. And despite all we have done, most women still find the experience of breast cancer profoundly isolating.

We can do more. At Living Beyond Breast Cancer, we do more by giving voice to the diverse experiences of women coping with breast cancer. The women who call our Survivors' Helpline, attend our conferences, visit www.lbbc.org and respond to our newsletters have varied feelings about their diagnoses. But they all want to share their story, with one person or with many, to process their experiences and possibly help others to do the same.

This remarkable book honors so many of the values and goals to which we aspire at Living Beyond Breast Cancer. As I read *Voices of Breast Cancer*, I was struck by how many of these thoughtful essays focused on relationships: a daughter whose greatest fear is sharing her diagnosis with her mother; a son remembering his mother's treatment when he was a child; a friend searching for words of comfort for a woman facing months of chemotherapy. In sharing their stories, these writers show breast cancer is a disease that touches both our genetic families and our "created" families—our friends, work colleagues, acquaintances.

These voices, and these stories, must be heard. Every time a woman shares her story, she gives voice to the powerful and unique experiences of people affected by breast cancer. She reminds us that breast cancer is not about pink ribbons or the small, incremental improvements we make each day in breast cancer care. It is about living and loving and caring for our communities, while also never abandoning the quest to find the causes and ultimately the cures for breast cancer.

Living Beyond Breast Cancer is a national education and support organization, the mission of which is to empower all women affected by breast cancer to live as long as possible with the best quality of life. Jean Sachs has served as the Executive Director of LBBC since 1996. During her tenure, LBBC has earned national recognition for the quality of its educational programs for a consumer audience. Each year more than 34,000 breast cancer survivors attend or participate in LBBC programs. In 1998 and 2003, GlaxoSmithKline honored Living Beyond Breast Cancer for best practices with its International Impact Award. LBBC is one of only two organizations in the Philadelphia region to receive this prestigious award twice.

Foreword

Alexander J. Swistel, M.D.

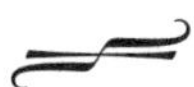

Breast Cancer. Few words are more devastating for a woman to hear. This year, over 200,000 women like my patient Debra LaChance, the creator of this wonderful book, will hear them. Forty thousand will die of the disease. The medical science community has tried with little success to understand why people get breast cancer. Patients ask, "Was it my lifestyle? Is it in my family? Should I have done something differently?" Sadly, there is no answer yet. But we do have encouraging news about the treatment of breast cancer to tell women like Debra. No longer must these women face the radical treatment and debilitating aftercare which often scarred them for life. We are finding this disease at an earlier, curable stage, fighting it with gentler, more effective treatments and improving survival rates. Major research continues at the genetic and molecular levels to find the cause and understand the mechanism of this disease. This important work, together with improved early detection, new surgical techniques and a multidisciplinary approach to patient care, is turning more patients like Debra into survivors.

For the first time in history, the death rate from breast cancer is in decline. While it may be true that the overall incidence of breast cancer is up, this statistic may simply be a reflection of "baby boomer" demographics at work. The boomer population has affected all aspects of life for a generation and this large bulge in the population is now entering the prime time of breast cancer diagnosis. The incidence of breast cancer is age dependent, in large part striking women in their late forties to early sixties, which happens to mirror the present age of the boomer population. But there is no doubt that the trend of improved survival will continue.

Yet despite our steady march towards understanding and eliminating or controlling the disease, we still have a long way to go. We have yet to see any change in the incidence of breast cancer in the younger, *premenopausal* or *perimenopausal* group. We need to make every effort to identify this disease in its earliest stage, since early detection will continue to be the key to greater survival rates for the near future.

Advances in early screening technology, including continuing improvements in mammography technology, the increasing role of breast ultrasound and a greater acceptance of and facility with the diagnostic power of *magnetic resonance imaging* (MRI), are helping identify the disease at a much earlier stage. Along with these advances, an increasing number of women are being made aware of the advantages of early screening and are following screening guidelines. As the number of women screened has increased, the number of newly diagnosed, small cancers has also increased, resulting in a substantial decrease in the size, and therefore the stage, of the cancer at the time of presentation. This decrease in size translates directly into improved curative survival and has resulted in the need for less radical treatment. There is little doubt that as newer imaging technologies appear, we shall continue to see the disease identified in ever-smaller amounts. Even now, most clinicians report that tumor registries are currently seeing a marked shift in the size of tumors reported into stages 0 and I, the earliest stages.

Surgical techniques continue to improve. Gone are the days of radical, disfiguring surgery. Today, the trend is towards *onco-plas-*

tic options, where the breast surgeon works closely with a plastic surgeon towards the dual goal of removing all of the disease and providing the patient with an excellent cosmetic outcome. Patients now worry less about how they will look after surgery as they move on with their lives. *Sentinel node biopsy*, a procedure for removing and testing the first lymph node to which it is believed breast cancer will spread, has eliminated many of the problems seen in years past with *lymphedema*, or swelling of the arm near where the affected nodes are found. New surgical techniques have less negative effect on post-surgery range of arm motion, and women are better able to resume normal activities and enjoy fulfilling lives. The other specialties involved in breast cancer treatment have also refined their techniques. For example, radiation oncologists are now actively seeking ways to perform extremely targeted irradiation, where not long ago whole breast radiation therapies were the standard. With less irradiation, patients do not have some of the side effects seen in the past, including the potential negative effect on the lungs and heart.

The increase in the survival rate is, in large part, based on some very important advances in drug therapies that have occurred just over the past 10 years. *Targeted therapies*, the use of new drugs or other substances to identify and attack specific cancer cells without harming normal cells, allow oncologists to tailor the dosages for the individual patient, resulting in fewer and less severe systemic side effects. An example is the drug tamoxifen, a potent antihormonal compound that has the ability to curtail breast cancer development. A recent trial testing the drug on women who had a high risk for developing breast cancer demonstrated that tamoxifen could safely prevent the onset or recurrence of breast cancer. It has become widely available and has shown a wonderful success rate in those women.

The rise of the comprehensive breast center has also resulted in major improvements in the delivery of quality care to breast cancer patients. That this disease requires a multidisciplinary approach became clear over the last 15 years and breast centers facilitate this process. Surgeons and radiation and medical oncologists all interact to discuss and present the best possible care to the individual. The breast center also brings the patient together with other important caregivers such as prevention groups, counselors and support groups organized around the specific needs of the patient, of younger patients concerned about fertility or older women concerned about severe menopausal symptoms secondary to treatments. Genetic counseling within the breast center setting has become increasingly important as we struggle to identify families with high numbers of members who are prone to develop the disease. Genetic studies allow doctors to explain various risk reduction strategies to family members who might test positive to a known breast cancer gene mutation. This risk analysis allows an improvement in survival and in the quality of the life of the patient and their families. The individual can obtain a better understanding of her overall risk and hence can attain some control over the previously inevitable consequence of developing breast cancer at some future date.

Understanding the mechanism of this disease will be the next great breakthrough in treatment. It is just around the corner. And as strange as it may sound, it is my hope and belief that soon I will never have to meet such wonderful people as Debra LaChance, at least not where I work.

Alexander J. Swistel, M.D. is the Director of the Weill Cornell Breast Center and a nationally renowned breast surgeon. A graduate of Harvard University, he received his medical degree from Brown University School of Medicine in 1975. He is Associate Professor of Clinical Surgery at Weill Cornell Medical College, Associate Attending at New York-Presbyterian Hospital's Department of Surgery and Section Chief of the Breast Service at the New York Cornell Center.

Dr. Swistel pioneered the use of new, less invasive treatment options for women with breast cancer. He developed an early protocol using laser-guided destruction of small breast tumors to minimize surgical intervention. He was the first surgeon in New York to perform a skin-sparing mastectomy, a revolution in the standard mastectomy procedure that, when combined with immediate reconstruction, provides a vastly improved cosmetic outcome and improved survival. Dr. Swistel was one of the first physicians in the state to employ sentinel lymph node biopsy to minimize axillary surgery. He continues to develop surgical methods combining effective tumor removal with reconstructive techniques that leave the patients without visible scars.

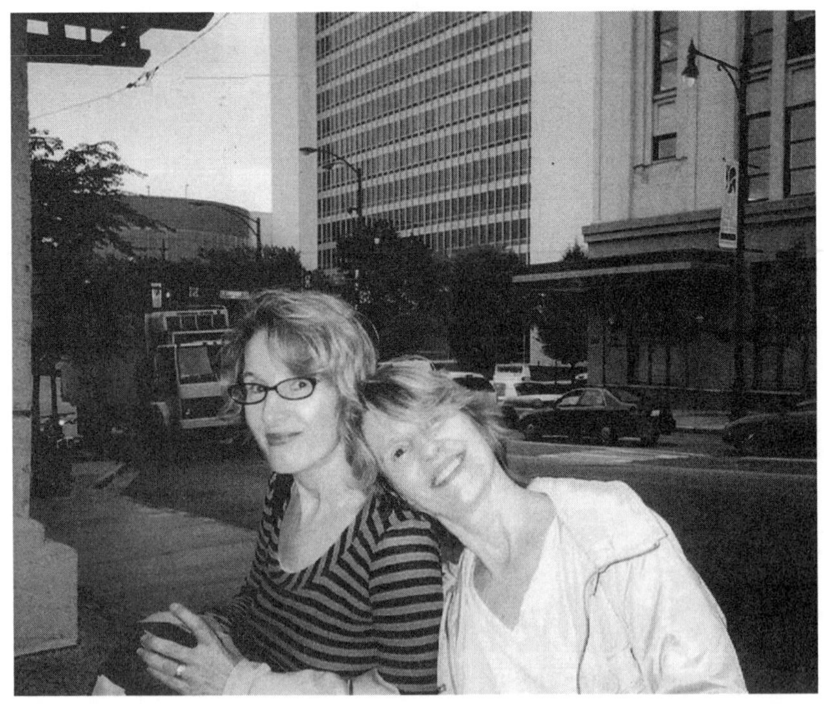

Denise and Debra LaChance

Introduction
The Healing Project
Debra LaChance

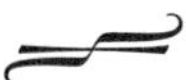

I wanted to ask the people around me, "Would you please raise your hand if you feel as isolated as I do?"

Walking the busy streets of Manhattan on a beautiful sunny day, I was surrounded by people but I'd never felt so alone. Just minutes before, my doctors had broken the news to me that I had a particularly aggressive form of breast cancer.

Since moving to New York from a small town in Rhode Island, I'd had my share of ups and downs but had always risen to the challenges that living and working in New York could bring. But on this summer afternoon, I felt as if the world was suddenly rushing past me while I moved in slow motion along the crowded sidewalk. It was the next step I knew I had to take that seemed to freeze me in my steps, the one I dreaded the most: how was I going to tell my twin sister Denise? How do you tell someone you love that you have cancer?

My sister and I are as close as only twins can be. Denise is my best friend, my greatest supporter, my closest confidante. Always at my side as I built successful businesses in fashion, technology, and real estate, we had faced challenges together in the past, but cancer was unknown territory. As I reached for my phone to make the call, I shook my head at the thought that I'd have several similar calls to make. Telling my loved ones I had cancer would be far worse than having heard it myself.

But with a life of love and support behind us and uncertainty ahead, Denise and I did what we had always done: we got to work. There was much to do and a short amount of time in which to do it: specialists to consult; doctors to interview; treatment plans to decide upon; hospitals to find. And the clock was ticking. The gravity of these tasks made my day-to-day business pale in comparison. This job wouldn't allow a day off.

Almost automatically, one of the first things I began to seek out, besides doctors, was a sense of connection. I needed to hear from others who had gone through what I was experiencing, who truly understood what it meant and who might be able to help. I wasn't ready for a regular support group and, with surgery and treatment looming, I simply didn't have the time. But I am an avid reader, and I assumed that finding the personal stories of those who had gone through this ordeal before me would be easy. But there seemed to be a vacuum; almost nothing. Where were the *real people* to talk to? Where was the literature that wasn't just about the "hardcore" science of the disease? I found just one book, *Just Get Me Through This—The Practical Guide to Breast Cancer*, by Deborah Cohen, that helped. It made me laugh and cry and pushed me onward down the road to acceptance of the diagnosis. But I knew there were countless others out there, just like me, who needed to tell their stories—and to hear the stories of others as well. I decided that part of my own, ongoing healing process would be to find a way to bring people like me together, to create some kind of forum where their stories could be shared.

But first I had to find the doctors who would make the physical healing possible. From the beginning, I knew I wanted a female surgeon to handle my case, but as Denise and I did the research about the disease and its treatment, one doctor's name kept repeating: Dr. Alexander Swistel, the Director of the Weill Cornell Breast Center at Weill Medical College at Cornell University. He wasn't in my insurance network, but after meeting with him I knew he was *the one*. Dr. Swistel put me at my ease, gave me confidence and made me feel that I was in good hands. I also felt instant rapport with my oncologist, Dr. Ellen Gold. Dr. Gold was frank and honest, while allowing me the room to share my feelings as time rushed by and my surgery loomed. I'm so thankful that my journey led me to these amazing doctors, who were so instrumental in my care and in demonstrating by example that caring is truly a big part of the healing process.

Besides my family, my doctors and my friends, what got me through that frightening process were the little lies I told myself to help me get my mind wrapped around the reality of my situation. I'd seen my pathology report, and I started to devour all the literature on the disease, selecting all of the information that would help me to put the best "spin" on my condition. There's so much information out there, so many statistics, reports and findings that I could always find something to latch onto that would allow me to continually push the scariest possibilities away.

But the initial pathology report was wrong. The corrected report I received soon after the first indicated the highest presence of HER2 (human epidermal growth factor receptor) in my tumor, which results in significantly lower survival rates because its presence can lead to an intense proliferation of cancer cells. Time stood still for me as I read this new report, and in that stillness I finally felt the full impact of my diagnosis. Denial stopped working. I knew I'd need chemotherapy. Like so many women, the thought of losing my hair to chemotherapy brought it all crashing home. Hitting that hard wall of reality, the time had come to finally face it and fight… or not.

I chose to fight, and in making that choice my vision of community crystallized and The Healing Project was born. My thoughts kept returning to that walk through Manhattan after I'd heard my diagnosis and that feeling of terrible loneliness. As sympathetic as friends and loved ones could be, I felt that no one could truly understand this journey except someone who had been through it themselves. As the day of my surgery drew closer, I became convinced that getting and giving courage, comfort, and strength were as important as good medical care. I became determined to help build a community for people like me who were undergoing the terribly isolating experience of dealing with a life-threatening disease. This would be *The Healing Project*'s mission: to become a bridge across which people can make those all-important emotional connections.

When the day of my surgery arrived, the hardest moment of the whole ordeal was when I had to leave Denise behind at the door of the operating room. But Doctor Swistel actually came out and walked me in. What a blessing. He even called me from his vacation later to check on how I was doing.

I had a second operation after the first failed to clear the margins of my cancer, then sixteen weeks of chemotherapy every two weeks followed by radiation, every day, for seven weeks. I didn't want to wait for my hair to come out in clumps so I went out and had my head it shaved. It gave me something else I could do for myself, rather than just sitting around and waiting. Staying as active, and as proactive, as possible was very important to me. Throughout the ordeal I didn't stop working and went about my life with as much zeal as my varying energies would allow.

Following radiation, my biomarkers indicated I was a candidate for the new drug Herceptin® which targets HER2 and which had shown remarkable success in patients with aggressive breast cancer. But since the first round of chemo had caused damage to my heart I needed to be monitored during the treatments. If good things come in threes, my cardiologist, Doctor Allison Spatz, was my third miraculous doctor. She paid close attention to my case, and when she went off my insurance plan in the middle of my treatments, she actually refused to take payment for her work! I ultimately took Herceptin® for a year with good results.

During chemotherapy, Dr. Gold encouraged me to explore alternative and complementary treatments, including herbal mixtures and vitamin supplements. I know some people don't believe in the holistic approach, but I want to believe it worked for me. My immune system was pumped up when it should have been down and I didn't get the flu like so many other people in New York that season. That's an important point about dealing with cancer: it comes down to what you choose to believe. There are so many people with so many opinions and there are so many variables to consider. Ultimately, you have to do what's right for yourself, realize that you're not as alone as you might feel, and seek out the people who know best what it's like to be you.

And those are the people I want to help me build *The Healing Project* community. In addition to my daily work during my treatments, I began to develop *The Healing Project* as a place where people can contribute funds for research, time for connecting with and mentoring others and, most of all, a place to share their stories. Since then, The Healing Project has been collecting stories by those touched by breast cancer and other diseases for books like this one: books that inspire and inform for the road ahead and impart a sense of community for those caught up in the moment. These books are meant to be an oasis where they can find strength in shared experiences.

In 2007, my mother was also diagnosed with breast cancer which has given *The Healing Project*'s mission an even greater urgency. My own breast cancer experience helped me navigate my mother through the process. And although she is truly a soldier in her own right, it was rewarding to be able to guide her thoughtfully down her path. She is doing well, and my experience on the caregiver side of the equation gave me a whole new perspective on what *The Healing Project* is all about and the positive impact it can have on people's lives.

In addition to the books, we're also working on other initiatives through *The Healing Projec*t, including *Voices Who Care* a "virtual support group" which will allow patients, their families and friends to connect with others in real time. I don't want anyone to have to feel the way I did that day of my diagnosis when I was walking through the city alone and afraid. There's so much strength in others—you just have to find them. I realize how fortunate I was to have people who were willing to give of themselves and their time. The healing begins with giving to others.

So *The Healing Project* is part of my own healing, a signpost on my road ahead. And looking ahead, friends ask me if I consider myself cancer free. I choose not to. "The Big C" gives me something tangible with which to create priorities for my life. So I view the experience of cancer as an opportunity, to develop my own list of "Big Cs":

To show Courage in the face of so much challenge.

To accept Caring as it comes.

To take Comfort from others.

To let yourself and others Cry.

To know it is OK to Complain.

To stay Connected with those you love.

To be Constant in your ability to rise above but never feel guilty when you can't.

To build Character for when you come out on the other side.

To Create kinship with others not as lucky as you.

To say I Can.

To say I Cannot.

To opt for Plan "C" if you must.

To take Control of your diagnosis and become your own advocate.

To believe in a Cure, if only for your heart.

To make Choices that you can live or die with.

Finally, with cancer you have to be ready to chart a new Course, for rest of your life, no matter what the outcome. And it helps to see that others are busy charting their own courses along with you. That's what these stories are all about. Reading these amazing contributions to the *Voices Of* series convinces me that I don't really have a remarkable story at all.

The truth is *everyone* does.

Debra LaChance is the creator and founder of The Healing Project.

Lessons in "Judo Biology"

Michael Shepard, Ph.D.

Two challenges have fed my lifelong passion as a molecular biologist and an entrepreneur in pursuit of advanced cancer drug therapies: understanding the seeming perversities of Nature and, in doing so, reducing the toxicities of chemotherapy.

While doing research at Indiana University on how bacteria develop resistance to antibiotics, I discovered that certain drug-resistant bacteria actually promote their own growth using the very antibiotics they were once resistant to. This was my first encounter with one of Nature's perversities and the first of the many lessons I would learn in what I call "Judo Biology."

Judo is actually comprised of two words, "Ju," meaning gentle and "Do," meaning way. The words describe a principle in martial arts by which a combatant yields to his attacker's energy so that the attacker's own force can be used against him. This principle is similar to one of the important characteristics of the "super bugs" we hear so much about today—bacteria that are difficult to kill, running amok and causing many difficulties for patients and health care professionals. I later learned that our own cells are adept at Judo Biology when they take a genetic miscue to grow uncontrollably into cancer.

One of the greatest challenges for a scientist studying chemotherapy treatment today is figuring out better ways to attack cancerous tumor cells without harming normal cells in the process. Most cancer drugs are quite toxic to normal cells and the dose that can be given to a patient is limited by this often-intractable fact. For instance, one of the most common cancer drugs is a compound called fluorouracil, or 5-FU. 5-FU is severely toxic to a quarter of the patients who receive the drug, requiring that these patients' treatment be stopped or that they receive additional medical intervention, with no guarantee of increased survival. The most common of these toxicities is diarrhea, but other adverse reactions, such as the suppression of the body's natural defenses to illnesses, can also occur. I turned to research in this area because it seemed to me that, in the 21st century, we ought to be able to do a lot better than this.

The invention of Herceptin® was the result of my work on the mechanisms of drug resistance and my goal of developing less toxic, more selective cancer therapies. While at the biotechnology company Genentech in the late 1980's, my research team found, to our surprise, that a newly discovered anti-cancer protein called *tumor necrosis factor*, or TNF, was only effective against one-third of the tumor cells on which it was tested. This was not what we had expected: previous studies indicated that this protein was effective against a much broader range of cancers. Further work on the problem by our team, together with Dr. Hans Schrieber at the University of Chicago, led us to discover that TNF was made by *macrophages* (a type of natural immune cell) when the macrophages came into contact with tumor cells. The macrophage would produce TNF that would kill the young, small tumor. As we continued our investigations we found that many types of tumor cells start out sensitive to the toxic effects of TNF, but then become resistant to it. Quite amazingly, we also learned that tumor cell growth was actually *stimulated by TNF*—a discovery almost identical to that made in my earlier research at Indiana

University, where we discovered that drug-resistant bacteria use antibiotics as nutritional supplements to grow. While the biochemical mechanisms of this "tumor judo" were and are still not completely understood, the clinical implications became very clear: something changed inside the tumor cells that prevented them from being destroyed by TNF.

As is often the case in the research community, something else happened in two other laboratories that had a big impact on my work and led directly to the invention of Herceptin®. UCLA's Dr. Dennis Slamon had begun research with Dr. Axel Ullrich, who was also at Genentech (working one floor above me), which showed that breast cancer patients who express large amounts of a cancer-causing enzyme, a protein called p185-HER2 (or HER2), had especially aggressive disease. My laboratory group began to pursue the hypothesis that this protein might also be responsible for tumor resistance to our TNF protein. By increasing the amount of HER2 in TNF-sensitive tumor cells, we were able to show increased resistance to the TNF anti-tumor protein. We also showed that we could reduce this resistance by treating the tumor cells with an antibody that partly neutralized the activity of HER2. Our work demonstrated that large amounts of HER2 protein help tumor cells become resistant to destruction by the body's immune system and that the anti-HER2 antibody could inhibit tumor growth as well as partly restore cancer cell sensitivity to TNF. We were learning how to apply Judo Biology against our foe.

During the early testing of Herceptin® I became acquainted with some cancer patients who agreed to participate in the drug's clinical trials. For the first time in my career I began to truly understand that it was one thing to find cancer a fascinating object of scientific study, and quite another to live with the disease. In the very first clinical study, it happened that one of our patients was supposed to return to the clinic within 48 hours after treatment for a follow-up examination. This was a critical time for the experiment because, as part of our proof that the antibody had a chance at working, we needed to prove it could concentrate itself in tumors that produced large amounts of HER2. The person didn't show up as scheduled. I was furious with this patient. I asked a fellow researcher what could possibly have happened. His answer was that the patient had decided it was more important to take her child to a soccer game than to return for the exam.

This event changed my life forever. It helped me to understand that if we can add just a few days or weeks to someone's life, they can take their kids to a few more soccer games, go fishing once more, or work contentedly in their garden. This, I realized, was the point to my life's work.

The average time to market from the initial discovery of a drug is *ten years*. Drug development is an amazingly complex, emotional, intellectual and even physically demanding process. It can involve working 24-hour days for sometimes weeks at a time. Families are left waiting on Thanksgiving and Christmas. The antibody that gave rise to Herceptin® was created Christmas Day 1988. It was finally approved by the FDA some ten years and millions of dollars later.

I have always been a scientist, and I wish to stay a scientist. But in order to convert our antibody from a novel discovery into an anticancer therapeutic, I had to convince Genentech's management to spend what turned out to be more than $100 million to develop it into a real drug that could help people. Now that Herceptin® sales are approaching $1 billion per year, this doesn't seem like such a lot of money. But from where Genentech stood in the late 1980's this was no small commitment for the new but growing company. Nevertheless, I chose to fight for the development of the drug. To say that I was, and still am, fairly naïve politically would be an understatement. Although I "burned many bridges," I learned that entrepreneurship is a group process and, not unlike the subjects of my research, I learned to deal with resistance and turn negative energy into positive results.

Inventors of new medicines work in academic institutions, in large pharmaceutical and in smaller biotechnology companies. Regardless of their environment, they will always need to be politicians as well as inventors. Otherwise, it is impossible to obtain the financial support to develop the drug you have invented. Many scientists find this "netherworld" between science and business impossible to navigate. The constant stress and emotional roller coaster of getting the financing needed for discovery and development can result in some of the best scientists giving up and "sticking to the bench," or even leaving science altogether. Within the biotechnology companies, where a significant portion of the science is now being done in support of new medicines, "venture capital" and so-called "angel investors"—wealthy individuals who invest in private companies—support most of the work. In these venture-funded enterprises, entrepreneurial scientists and business associates will attempt to carry out a dramatic series of experiments resulting in a billion-dollar product. Whether or not a company is funded depends on the scientist's ability to convince investors of the potential success of both the science and the enterprise. Each candidate product is compared with all the others with respect to whether it will work and whether it can actually be developed with the resources at hand. I have now been through several cycles of this process: at Genentech, where the competition was vigorous but where my efforts eventually gave rise to Herceptin®; at Canji, where we developed a therapy against cancer now approved for use in China and undergoing testing in the U.S.; and at my first start-up company, NewBiotics, where a new drug to treat colon cancer was invented and is presently in clinical testing.

Today, I am a co-founder of Receptor BioLogix, where we have discovered a new way to identify low-toxicity biotherapeutics to treat cancer and autoimmune disease. Our lead drug candidate is one we hope will address the large proportion of cancers that are not successfully treated with Herceptin®. But through all of this

I'm still a humble student, one who has learned that true success in Judo Biology is measured in getting those stricken by this terrible disease out to the soccer fields again.

Dr. Shepard is a founder of Receptor BioLogix, a California-based biopharmaceutical company focused on developing a newly discovered class of protein therapeutics called Intron Fusion Proteins™ (IFP™) to treat cancer, autoimmune, metabolic and other diseases. While at Genentech, he led the discovery and development of Herceptin® for the treatment of breast cancer.

The Healing Project

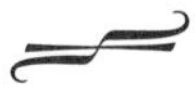

Individuals diagnosed with life-threatening or chronic, debilitating illnesses face countless physical, emotional, social, spiritual, and financial challenges during their treatment and throughout their lives. The support of family members, friends, and the community at large is essential to their successful recovery and their quality of life; access to accurate and current information about their illnesses enables patients and their caretakers to make informed decisions about treatment and post-treatment care. Founded in 2005 by Debra LaChance, *The Healing Project* is dedicated to promoting the health and well-being of these individuals, developing resources to enhance their quality of life and supporting the family members and friends who care for them. *The Healing Project* creates ways in which individuals can share their stories while providing access to current information about their illnesses and strives to promote public understanding of the impact such illnesses have on the lives of those affected. For more information about *The Healing Project* and its programs, please visit our website: www.thehealingproject.org.

Acknowledgments

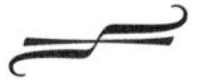

This book would not have been possible had it not been for the selfless dedication of many, many people giving freely of their valuable time and expertise. We'd particularly like to thank Theresa Russell and Amy Shore for their unending efforts to reach out to the people and organizations making so many contributions to this book; Lisa LaChance for her assistance with almost every aspect of this project; Melissa Marr for her invaluable assistance, insights and opinions; Drs. Alexander J. Swistel, Stephanie F. Bernik, Ellen Chuang and Malcolm Z. Roth for lending their extraordinary medical expertise; Drs. Allison Spatz, Elizabeth Beautyman, Desiree Clarke and Barbara Edelstein, all of whom, in their own way, made this book possible; and to the many, many people who submitted their stories to us, for their courage, their generosity and their humanity.

Part I
FINDING OUT

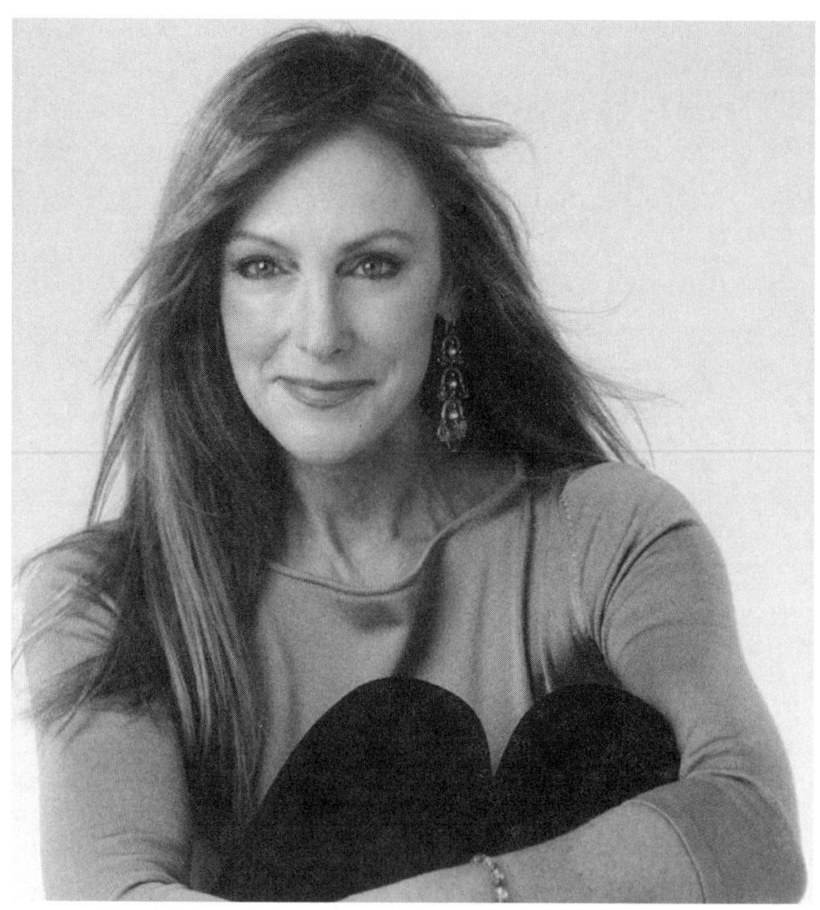

Peggy Fleming

Don't Wait

Peggy Fleming

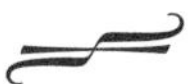

When I think back to 1998 and the month before I was diagnosed with breast cancer, I remember my main focus was on my family and broadcasting career. Oh, I was still performing a bit, but only in very special projects and very infrequently. I still had an 11-year-old son at home (my oldest son was off at college) and that, along with work, kept me from accepting much in the way of skating.

But I had accepted an offer from my friend, Robin Cousins, to skate in a Tribute to Hollywood show. Since I had been working out a lot (and my friend, Vera Wang, had offered costumes!), I said yes to skating in the show.

The month before the show, I was working at the U.S. National Championships for ABC when I found a small lump on my chest. I wasn't worried; I'd had a mammogram and checkup just five months earlier, and I had always been very consistent about annual exams, so this only slightly sharpened my radar. I knew that I should have it checked out, but I still wasn't concerned because of the fit lifestyle I had led for 50 years.

I ended up going to my doctor, seeing a breast surgeon, taking out the lump for a biopsy—all in the week before that performance, which I still managed to skate in.

Unfortunately, while I was away the results came back positive, and suddenly I was a breast cancer patient.

I'm so glad that my instincts sent me to the doctor with what I thought would be a minor thing. I thought the visit would just be for my peace of mind, but it opened up a big new chapter in my life. Early detection is the key to just about every serious illness out there. So many can be cured or their progress slowed considerably by today's advances in medicine. My treatment was not as difficult as it would have been had I waited and the disease progressed to a later stage. At my radiation treatments, I met many women dealing with cancers that were much farther along than mine.

And that is definitely my message as I travel around the country speaking to women's health groups and healthcare providers: don't wait.

I am so grateful to have caught my cancer early. I want to encourage others to give their heath the same attention. We all need to look at the big picture of our family health history, be aware of symptoms and changes in our bodies, and to share all this information with our doctors. My having breast cancer finally made my younger sister, Maxine, get her first mammogram at age 48, which fortunately was clear. Unfortunately, two years later she died of a heart attack, another major killer of women. She had ignored the early symptoms of heart disease. I think she would still be with us today if she had only gone to her doctor with those clues. Losing her was much more painful than my breast cancer. No matter the inconvenience and fear, being consistent with your checkups not only gives you peace of mind, it may uncover an early warning sign of a disease that, with today's medical treatments, can be treated with success.

Treatment did slow me down for a while, but it also kept me here with my family, to see my boys and now my grandsons grow up. I think that's a very fair trade.

Born and raised in San Jose, California, Peggy Fleming began skating at age 9 and quickly distinguished herself as an outstanding juvenile and novice skater. Developing a style marked not only by superb technical control but also by an exceptional sense of music and dance, Peggy came to dominate the women's skating competitions, becoming the U.S. Ladies Champion from 1964 through 1968, World Champion from 1966 to 1968 and finally winning the gold medal at the 1968 Olympics in Grenoble, France.

Soon after her win at Grenoble, Peggy starred in the first of five television specials and later toured for several years as a special guest star in the Ice Follies. She has been a commentator on figure skating for ABC Sports for the past 20 years.

Peggy was diagnosed with early stage breast cancer in 1998. Since that time, she has become a breast cancer activist who advocates for consistent examinations to ensure early detection and treatment.

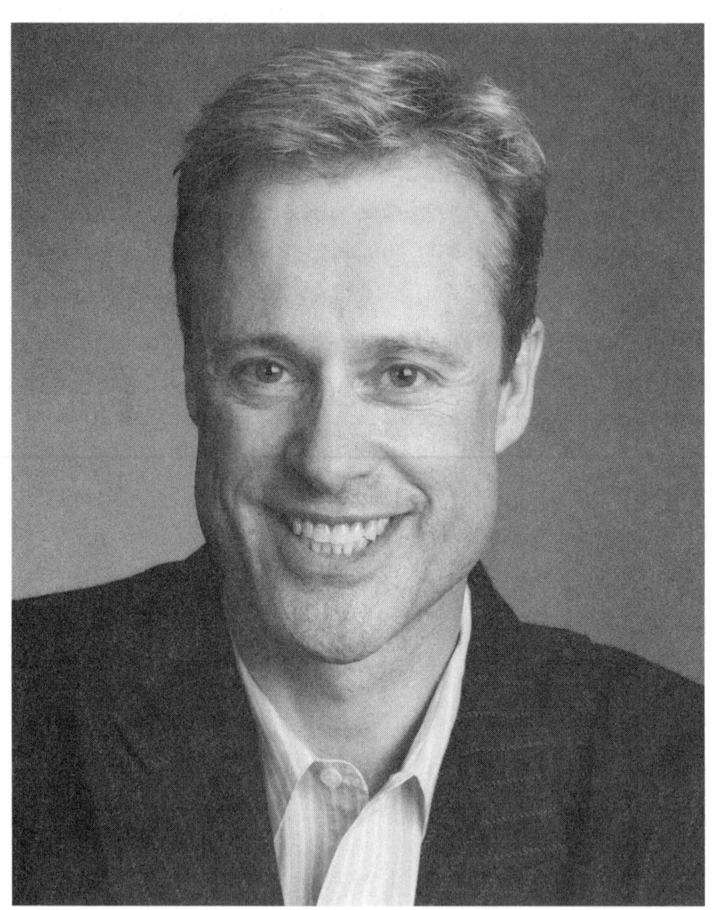

Glenn Connolly

The Bells of St. Patrick's

Glenn Connolly

As told to Richard Day Gore

You only turn forty once, and my Fortieth was going to be memorable. Ten days before my birthday, I decided to pull out all the stops with a big party in Manhattan. Friends. Co-workers. Champagne. Fun. Credit card in hand, I called the elegant St. Regis Hotel to book a dining room. Despite the short notice, they had one available and were more than happy to suggest catering options that would do the date proud.

But this wasn't to be just a vanity project. My birth date, December 17, has always been very special to me because it is also my mother's. We'd always celebrated together, until 1989, when she died of breast cancer. Now, as I looked ahead to this milestone, I felt the loss more deeply than ever. Her boy's Fortieth was something she'd always looked forward to, but thanks to breast cancer it was not to be. I decided this party wouldn't be just for me. As the champagne flutes were being raised in celebration of my birthday, I would propose an additional toast, to the memory of my mother, and I would ask my guests for donations to the Breast Cancer Research Foundation in her name.

My mother might have benefited from the Foundation's work, had it existed at the time of her diagnosis. When her cancer was found, in 1985, detection and treatment were far behind what medical science is capable of today. Her cancer was discovered, but too late to save her. It was a horrible experience, for her and for all of those around her. Mom was blessed with a fighter's toughness and she went through a radical mastectomy, chemo and the removal of 14 lymph nodes without losing her spirit. But it was hard, terribly hard. Science simply wasn't advanced enough to head off the disease's progress. Behind her smile she faded away slowly, painfully, relentlessly. It took almost four years for the cruel disease to finish its work.

Now here I was, several years later, planning a party that I hoped would be a fitting tribute to her courage. And maybe the money I raised might save someone from going through what she had endured. With my mother's struggle in my mind more than my birthday, I reserved a private party room and spared no expense.

A few hours after getting off the phone with the caterers, I was taking a shower, my mind spinning with the details of the upcoming party. As I washed, preoccupied with list-making, my hand passed over my left breast. And it stopped. Went back. Thoughts of decorations and guest lists melted from my mind as I felt a lump under my fingers. *A lump? Me? But I'm a man...* I could scarcely believe it, but there it was: hard, urgent and *real.* Like most other men, I might have ignored it if it hadn't been for my mother's history. Instead, I took a deep breath to keep myself from fainting.

I called my doctor the moment I stepped out of the shower. He told me to come in immediately. My day, which had begun with such pleasure, took an abrupt and chilling turn when, later that afternoon, the doctor referred me to a breast specialist with the warning that I shouldn't be surprised if I were told I would need a mammogram.

It was a couple of days until my appointment with the breast specialist, days during which my worry was constant. As positive as I tried to be, my thoughts kept turning back to those terrible years of my mother's decline. I couldn't banish the memories of her suffering. If it turned out to be the worst, I resolved that I wouldn't let myself go through what she had endured. I couldn't. The pain had been just too much.

Planning for the party, now looming ahead, gave me a little relief from my anxiety. During those days I shared my fears with only a few close friends, not wanting to make it seem more real by talking about it openly, not wanting to see all those frightened faces looking back at me. I was in constant dread. What if I had to make the unfortunate announcement at the St. Regis? That was not the memory of the event I wanted to send my guests home with.

My worries deepened when I headed for my appointment with the breast specialist at North Shore Hospital. North Shore was familiar territory to me. It was where my mother had gone for treatment. It's where she died. Back then, I would never have imagined that one day I'd be back as a breast cancer patient. But here I was, hearing the words my doctor had warned me of: I needed a mammogram. As we wrestled my scant flesh into the cold, hard and uncomfortable machine designed for a woman's breasts, the specialist tried his best to pull my mind from its funk. "You know," he said, "if this thing was supposed to look for testicular cancer, the guys who designed it would have made it velvet-lined."

But his effort to lighten my mood faded when he told me that the mammogram revealed a mass significant enough to warrant a sonogram. A few minutes later I had that procedure and in another few minutes I was told the mass would have to be removed for biopsy. For a moment my mind went blank as I tried to mentally process what was happening, then the reality of my situation crashed in around me as every fear came rushing into my mind. *How can this be?* Panic took hold of me for a moment, then the voice of grim logic. Wait, of course it can be. *Why not? Look at Mom...*

Look at Mom... That's just what I did. I took a breath and thought of her. I don't know what triggered it, perhaps survival instinct. But instead of thinking of my mother's suffering, I suddenly thought of her courage. While she had wasted away behind her smile, the smile itself had never wasted away. She had shown the power of the human spirit; for almost four years she had tapped into a strength no one knew she had and retained her sense of self. Sitting in the examination room, I turned away from my earlier resolve to avoid the suffering and vowed to fight.

So I put on a brave face when I saw the surgeon on the following Monday. I tried my best to smile and asked him, "Can they give me chemo that won't destroy my hair?" He was used to hearing this question of course, but not from a man. As I chatted with him about the surgery, bitter reality seemed to loosen its grip somewhat, allowing me to agitate over the upcoming party. It may seem shallow to worry about a party in light of what had happened, but I needed something else to focus on. The event was just a few days off. The surgeon sensed my urgency and scheduled the surgery as early as possible, for Thursday.

"How will I feel by Saturday?" I asked him. His silence indicated that the answer would depend on what the biopsy determined.

Thursday came, quickly. From the moment I'd found the lump, time had truly rushed by in a complete blur. In a little over a week it had swept me from doctor to specialist to surgeon and had finally thrown me into a cold, harshly lit operating room. The procedure was relatively easy, but everything was riding on what the biopsy would reveal. My father picked me up after the surgery. We were mostly silent on the drive home. His wife, my mother, had died at this very hospital. How many times had he made this same drive I wondered, as we drove away.

While the days leading to my surgery had rocketed by, now the hours dragged as I waited for the call about my biopsy results. Though now empowered by my mother's courage and my new resolve, I was still very scared and I tried to lose myself in getting ready for the party. But it was hard: mortality rates for male breast cancer are higher than for women, possibly because men are lax about checking themselves and less likely to take a concern to a doctor. I couldn't shake the terrible question: had I discovered the lump too late, as my mother had?

Friday came. The day before the party. The weather matched my mood: a cold winter day, rainy, with steel gray clouds hanging over the city. I was walking down Fifth Avenue to meet some friends for dinner, which, under the circumstances, I didn't want to do, when my cell phone rang. Its buzzing snapped me from my swirling thoughts and I realized that I was just then walking past St. Patrick's Cathedral. It was the doctor calling. My heart froze. My shoulders clenched. As he began to speak I looked at the towering cathedral and mouthed a prayer.

It was answered.

No breast cancer, just a lipoma, a benign fatty cyst.

I nearly collapsed in utter relief. I hung up the phone and exhaled a breath that seemed to have been held in tense suspension for weeks. As I strolled down Fifth Avenue to my date with my friends, I felt myself smiling for the first time in many days. I would tell them about my ordeal over dinner. I wondered, with another smile, if they would believe me when I told them that, when I hung up the phone from the doctor, the bells of St. Patrick's had begun to ring. They did ring, a thunderously beautiful song, and I'll always treasure the sound.

Saturday night arrived, and the staff at the St. Regis outdid themselves. The hotel was decorated for the holidays, and the party room was lighted with candles reflecting off the crystal glasses. The table centerpiece was a Christmas tree adorned with pink ribbons, in honor of my mother.

My guests were in a festive mood. When it came time for the toast, there was a collective gasp as I told them of my close call with breast cancer. It was only then, when I had broken the news, that the immense weight of what I had just brushed up against truly hit me. I realized my good fortune at having been given this opportunity to live, an opportunity that had been denied my mother.

My friends were moved as much by the tributes to my mother as by the holiday spirit, and were very generous in their contributions to the Breast Cancer Research Foundation. The party ran a couple of hours beyond what I had booked, but the hotel was in the spirit too, and let us stay on, free of extra charge.

Though it had been years since Mom passed, I felt very close to her on my fortieth birthday. In fact, it felt like she was with me at that party. I had narrowly escaped a sad walk in her shoes, and now, as the celebration went on around me, I knew that she was still walking with me.

Glenn Connolly resides in New York City where he works as a vice president with Sotheby's International Realty. For many years he has been an active supporter, board member and fundraiser for a number of charitable causes in the New York area, including Abilities! (formerly known as the National Center for Disability Services), the New York City chapter of PFLAG, the Breast Cancer Research Foundation and, most recently, Only Make Believe, an organization that brings an interactive theater experience to children confined to hospitals. He also supports the work of The Hetrick Martin Institute and Broadway Cares/Equity Fights Aids.

A Virginia native, Richard Day Gore came to New York City to pursue the arts. After lengthy forays into the fashion industry, he returns to the arts as Editor at LaChance Publishing. He is a cancer survivor.

Amazons Go Shopping

Mary E. Black

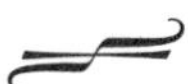

We are a family of one-breasted women. Some of us have none. Mine are in pretty good shape and have been widely admired in the past. Still are, my husband would say if asked. Good, functioning breasts, you could say, with almost four feeding years racked up on their odometer (lactometer?). Chances are they will not be with me forever: breast cancer runs in my family.

Sometimes I wonder which one will get lopped off first: the right one, which has always been a bit lumpy, or the left one, which was the children's favorite and so a bit bigger than the right, even now. "Because you were closer to my heart," I used to tell my two children when they asked me why, as babies, they liked feeding from my left breast the most.

We are also a family of matter-of-fact, overachieving women. Careers and medals and babies and ample breasts. So I have sensibly and unemotionally accepted that my breasts may be time-sensitive parts of my body. I check my breasts regularly using the latest techniques and my mammograms have been more or less on time. As a doctor, I have lived with cancer in all its shades, sharing the experience with my patients and my friends as well as with my family; I hold cancer in awe but not in terror. If you get cancer, you deal with it and move on.

But recently I have been quite shaken. What disturbs me greatly is genetic screening and the new option of surgery in advance of disease. Genetic screening adds a new variable. It inserts science and a percentage of risk into my carefully balanced and accepted beliefs. Genetic screening can tell me about my 11-year-old daughter's chances, and even her chances of passing it on to her daughters in turn. This is new territory for me, and I am not at all sure of my ground.

My insecurity began when my mother had her right breast off three years ago at the age of 77. She is a pragmatic and methodical doctor too, and we went through it together. Her surgery went well; together we monitored the functioning of the drain, the healing of the scar, the lymph node staging (no spread); we reviewed the histology (slow-growing squamous cell, nothing too scary), the tumor markers (estrogen receptor positive) and her various treatment options (tamoxifen, which she has now discontinued). We went shopping for prostheses together, weighing our options carefully—literally—as heavy prostheses can inflict shoulder ache on small, thin frames. We emailed to and fro, sorted out warranties, and when I finally persuaded her to go swimming I knew that both the physical and mental wounds were healing well. I had it all under control. The children and I checked my mother's scar as it went from red and raw to healed and pink. We juggled the various prostheses. The children saw that Grandma was just the same as ever and learned that it is not a catastrophe to remove a breast.

Then the hospital sent me a leaflet. Given our family history, genetic screening was strongly recommended. I shifted the leaflet from purse to drawer and back again. Now I had to choose: how much did I really want to know about my risk and the risk facing my daughter?

"Learn from the Amazons," my mother told my daughter. "My breast did its duty and fed your mother and although I miss it, I do not need it now."

We looked up Amazons on the Internet; mostly myth with some facts. From an early age Amazons were trained in the art of war, and the right breasts of young Amazon girls were removed and cauterized by their mothers so that the young warriors would be unimpeded, deft with their various weapons. My children and I were skeptical about some practices of this strictly matriarchal society: males were of no use to them other than for mating and as slaves; their limbs were amputated so that they could not rebel and escape; male babies were either given away at birth to neighboring tribes or killed. My daughter and I agreed that we liked Daddy and her brother (aged 6) and decided to keep them for the time being. We also agreed on this: Amazons discard their breasts if necessary.

Then I realized what was bothering me. I had accepted our family history, but only conditionally: to me, breast cancer was something that might happen when you became an old woman, only after your breasts had done their job. I had an unvoiced but unquestioned belief that young women in our family would not get breast cancer. But genetic counseling could prove me wrong. If we had certain genes, then we might be at risk for earlier cancer. I could barely accept this myself, so how could I ask an 11-year-old to face this possibility when her breasts had only recently started to grow? This was new ground and it involved fears—some buried, some that I could not speak of.

What made me finally book my appointment? A mixture of my medical training, a rigorous review of the facts and acceptance that new information might bring a difficult choice. But what prompted me most of all was the realization that I was behaving like an ostrich. I want to know as much of the truth as I can, and my daughter has the right to know, too.

So today I sit with my completed family history form, which I will send to the genetic counseling clinic. I have filled in the data about the single- and no-breasted women in our family tree: my grandmother, my two aunts, my mother, my first and second cousins. I am named in the family tree too, along with my sister, my nieces and my daughter. My daughter's appointment is marked on our family calendar; she will come to London with me for the day. After the appointment, we will have lunch at one of those Japanese restaurants where the dishes go round on a little railway track and then we will go clothes shopping. I will buy something low-cut and glamorous. My mother will send her best wishes and encouragement. Over the past year she has given up her prosthesis entirely and goes around a bit lopsided, but she takes the view that not many people look at your chest when you are 80, anyway. She also takes the view that no one will look at your chest if you are dead.

My daughter, in a fashion typical of the women in our family, takes a pragmatic view of our planned day out: in her opinion, modern-day Amazons should just get on with all the hospital stuff and then concentrate on shopping.

A graduate in medicine from Trinity College, Dublin, Mary E. Black trained in general medicine and infectious diseases in England and then moved into public health. She obtained a master's degree in International Health Policy and Management from Harvard's School of Public Health.

Her career has included over a decade of work with WHO and UNICEF in Bosnia and Herzegovina, Serbia, Croatia and other Balkan countries. She held a foundation chair of Public Health with the University of Queensland, Australia and established a new medical school based in Far North Queensland. She is the Royal College of Physicians' international advisor in Serbia and is currently President of the Harvard Club of Serbia. She is also a regular columnist for the *British Medical Journal*.

After Dr. Ozren Tosic saved her life from pirates in the Bay of Bengal, she married him. They have two children and currently live in Belgrade, where Dr. Black consults and teaches at Belgrade University.

Worrying Myself Well

Helen Kinrade

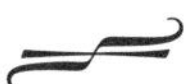

It's a cliché, but finding a lump in your breast that wasn't there last time you checked and which lingers after the premenstrual tension subsides is surely every woman's nightmare. That's where I found myself a few weeks ago, faced with the gnawing disquiet that goes along with discovering a lump and not having a team of experts on hand to tell me that everything is okay, that it's not one of *those* lumps.

I found it while in bed one night. As I turned, drowsy from sleep, onto my right side, something close to my armpit seemed to anchor my left breast into a more perky position than usual. Sleep fell away as I wrestled my right arm from beneath me to investigate the area and found a lump, largish and painful to the touch, on top of my pectoral muscle. "What the bloody hell is that?" I thought. After much shifting into different positions, plagued with apocalyptic visions of headscarves, I finally drifted off to sleep, consoling myself that I was imagining things and that it would be gone in the morning. Fortunately, after a couple of days, it was gone. Unfortunately, it had been replaced with burning pain, swellings that I'd never felt before, and enlarged milk ducts and glands.

I went to see the doctor, a woman not renowned for her lightness of touch. She elicited three loud yelps of pain from me as she examined my breast, and she promptly referred me to the breast clinic. "There's something there but there's no palpable lump, so I'm just going to put you in as a non-urgent case," she said, as I adjusted myself. "They'll probably be calling for you in the new year." I left in a daze. While I sat in my car, trying to take it all in, my sister rang to moan about the conditions of a new job she'd been offered. Now, I'm normally sympathetic to my sister's job plight. On this occasion though, I snapped back at her that I was late for work. For once, I had worries of my own that exceeded hers.

As the days progressed I got angry about the doctor's casual attitude. Her examination, while painful, was cursory. What if she'd missed something? What if I had cancer and it had been left to develop for the six weeks before the New Year? I tried to keep a sense of perspective. I couldn't stop this nagging cycle of worry but I kept it to myself, just letting friends and family in on the facts of the matter. Of course, their minds worked overtime too, but by and large we all kept things bottled up, because let's face it: that's the way it's done over here.

The big day arrived sooner than expected, around four weeks after my initial consultation. On the morning of the breast clinic appointment I told myself that I was feeling fine, relaxed. I tried to ignore my right hand as it clenched and unclenched involuntarily. I'd put on my heavy walking boots rather than heels for the appointment. I suppose it had something to do with a need to feel grounded, stable and secure because, strong woman that I am, I'd chosen to attend my appointment alone. I find it hard to accept support in times of stress; I'm the kind of person who likes to tend to her own wounds. Besides, I felt that my mum and sister, who'd both offered to join me on the day, would only bother me. So my heavy old boots came to the rescue, the kind of support that wouldn't try to feign breeziness or chat away to disguise the fact that they were worried and on the brink of tears. Even the nice, friendly ladies on the welcome desk got on my nerves as I walked into the hospital reception: poor unsuspecting buggers. I could scarcely bring myself to look one old lady in the eye as she told me where the breast clinic was.

I'd come prepared for a long wait and I wasn't disappointed: over an hour elapsed before my name was called. Then I was in the examination room, naked from the waist up, apart from a blue paper cape which seemed a waste of time considering that it was pushed aside a nanosecond after the consultant entered the room, heralded in from behind a curtain by Sue, the breast nurse. Quite an entrance, I'd thought as they paraded smartly into the room. I had mental images of him at home, marching into his dining room at tea time from behind velvet curtains. The consultant was very nice and a lot gentler than my GP had been. I was able to say "Er, that's tender just there," as he probed an area of my armpit that had elicited a "yee-ow" when my GP had grappled with it earlier.

I had expected the specialist to tell me that everything was fine and that I was worrying over nothing—silly I suppose, considering that I'd been referred to him in the first place, but I was genuinely taken aback when he told me he was going to send me to X-ray for a mammogram. I was handed a little envelope to give to the X-ray receptionist and, dressed again, I set off down the corridor. As I walked I started to think about my decision to come to this appointment alone, and I had my first conscious sense of foreboding. I allowed myself to think about the possibility that the news could be bad and that I was about to be told that I had cancer. I began to feel like a bloody idiot for not asking someone to come along with me.

Another hour and a half elapsed as I sat in the X-ray waiting room. Eventually a nervy, harassed-looking nurse called my name and ushered me down the corridor towards the mammography suite. She cracked a few nursing gallows-humor jokes as we walked. A fellow nurse would have smirked, probably.

The waiting area was papered in an attempt to make it look like someone's living room. Inside the suite I was asked to strip to the waist in an adjoining cubicle and I soon emerged, wearing another paper cape. So dressed, I sat with three other nervous women who, like me, were be-caped and waiting either for a mammogram or to be told they'd need to have an additional ultrasound. Waiting with me initially was a nicely spoken, well-groomed mature lady who was clearly frightened about what she was about to be told. I sat and listened as the nervy nurse went on and on to the woman about how stretched facilities were on the Isle of Man and how we should be grateful for the quality of service we have over here. I realize that the life of a breast screening nurse must be grim and bloody depressing; but this didn't assuage a nagging desire to tap her on the arm and suggest that she might want to talk a bit less and listen a bit more. But then, I'm not a breast nurse. I'm sure they need to inure themselves against a daily tidal wave of fear and despair.

The mammogram took place in a small room with subdued lighting. The machine was tall, all beige enamel and Plexiglas. In a strange and alarming way, my first impressions of the plates that supported the breast and squashed it down reminded me of the meat slicer at the deli counter of the supermarket I'd worked in as a teenager. A nurse helped me shuffle this way and that, in order to get into position for each of the four scans. The downwards compressions were fairly straightforward for me and only briefly uncomfortable. The sideways compressions were less comfortable, although this was mainly due to the strange contorted position that I had to stand in; akin to yoga but with added radiation.

Again, it was all over in a moment. All in all, the mammogram, surprisingly, was just the way it had been described in the information leaflet I'd received in the mail: uncomfortable, a little strange, but okay. Not the "titty-mangle" that one of the ladies waiting outside for their scans told me about when I emerged, and which elicited the first proper laugh out of all of us that morning. Flicking through an old copy of *Heat* magazine, we spotted the enormous, naked, saggy-boobed characters out of "Little Britain" and we all had another good laugh about how on earth they'd get tits that saggy to stay on the base-plate of the mammogram equipment. The other woman waiting with us, a pretty, scarlet-haired woman, said that this is how her tits had looked after they'd been through the mangle and we all collapsed laughing again. It felt good to laugh. Maybe the presence of the saggy-boobed Little Britain characters was the reason why that magazine had stayed in the waiting room all year.

Then the nervy nurse reappeared, ready to give us the preliminary results of our mammograms. It didn't take a genius to deduce that if we were told we could get dressed and get our results from the breast consultant then the news was good and that if we were told we should wait in order to have an ultrasound then the news might be bad. The nurse beamed a joyless grin at me and the woman who'd made the titty-mangle joke. "Okay," she said to the titty-mangle joke woman, "you can go and get dressed because your results are ready." I saw the woman's shoulders relax at the news. "And you," she said, pointing at me, "need to come with me to have an ultrasound." A cold dread started to creep over me. I started to gather my things.

"Oh, hang on," the nurse interjected, "I think I might have got that the wrong way around hahaha!" The three of us women cast looks at each other, then looked up at her. If nothing else, the nurse needed a holiday. She disappeared out of the room and returned a few seconds later. "Okay, I got it the wrong way round hahaha," she said. The woman who seconds before had thought everything was all okay paled slightly and followed her out for an ultrasound. I watched them go and went into the cubicle to get dressed.

When I emerged from the cubicle I was alone. I had to gather up my things and wait to be called. I'd been given a laminated card, which I needed to hand to reception at the breast clinic and the card slipped out of my hands. I bent over to retrieve it. Just then, the nervy nurse reappeared. Faced with my (clothed) arse as I bent over the chairs, she began to laugh uncontrollably. "Oh, haha-haha, I wasn't expecting to see that! Hahahahaha!" I smiled wanly and played along. "Yup, you don't get many of those to the pound," I said. The nurse continued to laugh and laugh. I'd had enough. I looked her in the eye. "It's not that bloody funny," I said. She stopped laughing, finally, and gave me directions to the breast clinic.

When I returned to the breast clinic it was empty. A trio of nurses stood chatting down the clinic's corridor. I caught their eyes and one of them motioned that she would be down to see me in a moment. Her casual nature told me what I needed to know as she ushered me into the examination room: I knew I didn't have cancer. The consultant swept in once again from behind the curtain and, looming over me, told me happily that I was absolutely fine. "What about the lumps in my breast?" I asked. "Oh, take evening primrose oil," he said. "Oh, but I do," I said, "I've been taking it for over ten years." "Well, keep doing it."

That was that. No explanation for my symptoms. No further examination. I got the feeling that if it wasn't cancer, this doctor wasn't interested. I supposed that was fair enough.

Another month has passed. I've still got pains, lumps and sensations—in both breasts now—but at least I know they're not cancerous. As to what is causing them, well, your guess is as good as mine. I'm taking extra evening primrose oil and hoping for the best. Apparently there's a new buzzword in the medical profession for people like me: the "worried well." It seems that thanks to people like Kylie Minogue, women are flocking to our GPs, wanting to get benign lumps and bumps checked over and the medical profession is trying to find the best ways to keep us away from their resources. In a bleak way, I suppose this is comforting. I can shrug away the next burning sensation when it comes, forget about any lumps that come but don't stay. I've been told that I'm well, and I'm doing my best not to worry.

Helen Kinrade left a career in cognitive neuroscience research in order to return to her birthplace, the Isle of Man. She stays sane by writing about how she's adjusted from her old life to the new, and an administration job keeps the wolf from the door. She's single but hopeful.

Breast Cancer: What Every Woman Should Know

Stephanie F. Bernik, MD, FACS

One in eight women will develop breast cancer during the course of their lifetime, making it, after skin cancer, the most common cancer in women. Although breast cancer primarily affects women, men can also develop the disease, albeit at a much lower rate. In 2006, there were over 175,000 cases of breast cancer and over 40,000 people died of the disease. Most people tend to think it is found only in older women, but it afflicts both the old and the young. In fact, breast cancer is the leading cause of death in women ages 15–59 and one in 229 women between the ages of 30 and 39 will develop breast cancer within a 10-year period.

What is breast cancer? Most breast cancers originate in the cells that line the *lobules* and *ducts* of the breast. The *lobules* are the glands where milk is produced and the *ducts* are the tubes that carry the milk out to the nipple. Breast cancer begins when one cell *mutates*, or undergoes an alteration in its genetic framework, or DNA, and starts growing and dividing rapidly and in a disorderly fashion. Cancer cells do not respond to the normal signals the body uses to regulate cell growth. Cancer cells drain the nutrients that normal cells need to survive, overgrow their boundaries and crowd out normal cells. They often form a mass, or *tumor*, that can invade surrounding tissue and potentially spread to other parts of the body.

The majority of breast cancers arise from the cells that line the ducts and are called *ductal carcinomas*. A cancer originating from the lobules is called *lobular carcinoma*. When a cancer is contained within the ducts of the breast it is called *ductal carcinoma in situ* (DCIS). This cancer is considered *preinvasive*, insofar as it has not spread from the ducts into the surrounding breast tissue, and the survival rate of patients with DCIS is excellent. *Lobular carcinoma in situ* (LCIS) is not actually a true cancer, but an abnormal overgrowth of the lobular cells contained within the lobules. The presence of LCIS in a woman's breast indicates that she has a significantly increased risk of developing a breast cancer in the future. An *invasive cancer* is one that has broken through the ducts or lobules and has started growing in the surrounding tissue. Invasive cancers are most often ductal (80%) or lobular (15%). At some point in their development, some cancer cells obtain the ability to travel from the breast to other parts of the body (*metastasize*) and grow in a new area.

Continued on page 34

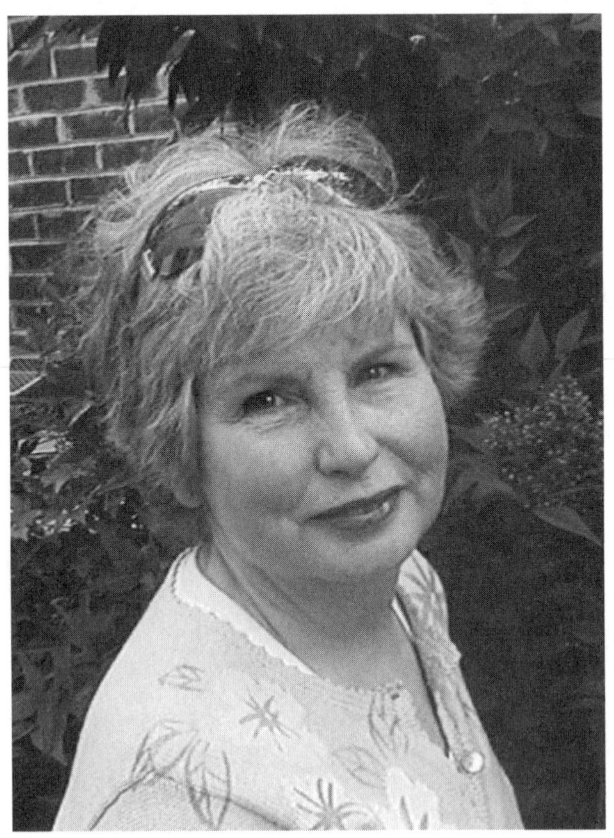

Janice A. Farringer

Biopsy

Janice A. Farringer

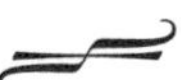

The suspense is not killing me, but it is interesting to see how all this is playing out over time. Last week I was going for the routine, yearly annoying-but-boring mammogram. This week I have had a long wire inserted into a body part, radiographed until I'm sure I am glowing (though they assure me I'm not), and have finally been told to go home and wait for a telephone call. A telephone call! I think that is pretty impersonal, crude even, but then, what insurance company will pay for an office visit "just to talk"?

So I was in the suspended time between being frightened and not knowing whether I should be really frightened. Cancer is not something I want to think about right now but here it is, the possibility. Then again, I may be overreacting, like when I left town before the impending hurricane last year. Nothing happened here because the darn thing turned and maybe this will be the same. Who knows?

The pathologist presumably would know by very late this afternoon; too late for a call. He or she will read the slides made from my "stuff" and will spend what, maybe five minutes, looking around that minute universe for stray terrorist cells. Cells that a week ago no one knew I might have. "Might" is the operative word. Maybe.

On the strength of maybe, I weekended with my innermost fears, ate nothing after midnight Sunday and got a friend to drop me off at the door of the ambulatory surgery clinic. I live not far from a major, major university medical center. Their new ambulatory clinic looks like a corporate architect was given the wrong assignment and too much money. I wondered at the marble and glass and soft carpet. The lighting was beautiful and the sweep of the check-in counter probably cost a couple acres of endangered rain forest.

I was checked in with a bar-coded bracelet and sent out to wait for a van to take me back across the street to Mammography at the older clinic building. I had been there for a whole day last week. I knew it well. Same routine: put on the gown, bag the clothes, sit here, wait. But this time there was a more delicate procedure to look forward to: the dreaded guide wire.

A very nice German resident actually stayed with me for the more excruciating parts. These involved compression and needles while reclining on your side with your elbows covering your face and your hands reaching for something to hold on to that isn't there. Try making conversation while doing that for half an hour. We did, though. When I got ready to leave I said, "Thank you." He searched for the right rejoinder and started with, "My pleasure." That didn't sound right to him and he sputtered "No problem" as he closed the door.

So now I'm wearing a long white gown over my black pants, in a wheelchair because of the wire that is sticking out of my left breast and with a gauze bandage under my gown. I must look odd with my plastic bag of clothes and my purse in my lap. Next thing I know, draped around my shoulders is another flat sheet, the better to hide my predicament and ward off street germs, I guess. I am wheeled down two floors and left at the valet parking entrance while a van is called. It takes awhile. I have visions of the OR staff pacing back and forth while in the background ka-ching, ka-ching makes a melody for the insurance company. We are all waiting on an $8.00 an hour van driver who decided to take a coffee break. Ka-ching.

Finally, my chariot arrives. I alight from the chair, arrange my toga and step into the van. The short drive is painless but slow. I step down and enter the marble and glass surgery center with what dignity I can muster given my bags and rumpled toga. I announce my arrival by holding out my bar code. Then, I grandly sweep to the public restroom to deal with all that fabric, among other things. I fold and tuck and toss in the mirror. I think I resemble Electra when I emerge. The rest is pretty grubby. I had only local numbing though it was a full-scale surgery. My fear of hurling was greater than my fear of being awake during the procedure. In fact, the whole team and I had a nice discussion of who was going to win the million dollars on *Survivor*. Everyone had an opinion. My physician, a young man in whom I have implicit trust, was chatty and casual. It was like someone else lying there. Recovery was uneventful, as my chart notes surely say.

So I'm home and it is two days later and I'm sore where all the bruising is. I've had a couple of Tylenol and one or two of the stronger pills. My family has called, friends brought me soup. Now it is me and me and me and myself and the waiting. Mostly I want to know what is next. Maybe nothing. I hope nothing. But a tiny part of me wants all this to result in something. You know? Not necessarily something bad, just some final thing. Maybe a statement that I'll never have to go through this again; I'm clean forever; no possibility of cancer. I know it won't be like that. Whatever the answer, I will not be able to forget. I'll pick up the telephone tomorrow and my life won't be the same. Yeah, I'm scared. One foot in front of the other is my motto and that is what I am sure I will do.

But I am temporarily suspended from my world. I have been working but it seems silly. Sorry, boss, but there are life and death things going on out there. Out there, over there, all those medical folks made me part of their world. The technicians, receptionists, physicians, lab techs, my German friend, the scrub nurses, they will be doing this medical stuff next week and the next, and the next. I only had to do it once, but it has messed me up. I'm lonely for that crowd. I want them to gather around me and tell me they did their best and that I'm okay. A smile, a joke maybe. What I have is the waiting… for a telephone call, a distant voice.

Janice Farringer is a six-year breast cancer survivor, a graduate of Vanderbilt University with a law degree from the University of Memphis, and works as a freelance writer in Chapel Hill, North Carolina.

Choice

Patricia Murray

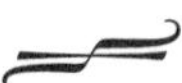

I will never win the lottery, see an alien spaceship or get attacked by a black bear. What are the chances? And although the odds are much better—about one woman in eight—I never thought I'd get breast cancer. Not me.

Why me? I stopped smoking after college. I practice yoga, donate to charity. I buy breast cancer research stamps at the post office when they have them. I've been a runner for thirty years; I ran the Boston Marathon twice. I eat fish. I don't drink nearly as much as I want to. I never lose at Monopoly.

On the flip-side, I cheat at Monopoly, eat entire bags of popcorn, speed on the turnpike. I scream and holler when the boys come home smelling like beer. My favorite word is fuck. I haven't washed the upstairs bathroom floor since last summer. I keep a joke going until it irritates, hold a grudge, enjoy gossip. I re-gift, buy clothes I don't need, lie to my kids about my past: *I never inhaled. Studied every Saturday night. Always told my parents the truth.* I lie about my age and I need to lose ten pounds. I screen phone calls. And my faith is eroding like beachfront property.

Good or bad, I didn't cause my cancer. I had no choice: cancer came uninvited. But I do have choices about my treatment, my attitude and my future. When it came, I read everything I could. I talked to other women. I chose the Breast Care Center in Scarborough, a hundred miles from home, rather than local treatment with a general surgeon who "does everything." Lumpectomy followed by six weeks of radiation. That was the plan.

When an MRI showed more cancer, I wrapped myself in grief and crawled into bed for days. Finished off the painkillers, read, napped, then read some more. Cried so hard I couldn't breathe. Then I wrote, scribbled really, down to the razor-sharp edge of my own mortality. Touched the cold, still face of it, then wrote some more.

On the third morning, I opened the shade. The room brightened. I jumped to the mirror; I was intact. I opened the window and inhaled the new day. Down in the kitchen, Ed poured my coffee. Kee needed help finding his baseball uniform. Devin needed a ride home after practice. Luke needed money. How did they know this was just what I needed?

Drove Kee to school.

"You're better now?" he asked, as he twisted the straps of his backpack.

"The worst part is over," I said.

That was the truth of it: I had traveled inward, touched the eerie stillness of fear and death, and came back.

Back home. Despite a forecast of rain, I put on two bras, wrapped my scarred breast with an ace bandage, and laced up my running shoes. Wild daffodils grew along the dirt road. The sweet scent of spring made the world clean. The call of peepers in the pond, the rush of water, the squawk of blue jays; the heartbeat of spring. Breathing deeply, the ecstasy of movement, of loving, of being loved, I was alive in my joy.

Dark clouds rolled in on a strong wind. The sky opened. I stripped off my hat, my jacket, stood in the road, face toward heaven. I held my left breast and I cried. On a road three miles from home I came to a balance between joy and sorrow.

Patricia Murray is a writer, teacher, mother of three and a breast cancer survivor. A recipient of a master's degree from the University of Maine, she resides in western Maine with her husband, sons and their dog.

Continued from page 25

What Causes Breast Cancer?

While the exact cause of breast cancer is unknown, it is generally believed that many factors play a role in its development. Environment, genetic predisposition, diet and activity level can all affect a person's risk of breast cancer. Most researchers feel that exposure to the hormone *estrogen* can increase the risk of breast cancer; therefore, since estrogen is naturally produced by the body, the greatest risk factor is *simply being a woman*. Women who are exposed to estrogen for a longer than average period of time (for example, a woman who gets her first menstrual cycle before the age of 12 or goes through menopause after the age of 55) can be at increased risk for breast cancer. It has now been shown that *combination hormone replacement therapy* (estrogen combined with progesterone), taken to relieve the symptoms of menopause, also increases a woman's risk of breast cancer, again due to increased exposure to estrogen. Birth control pills, another form of estrogen introduced to the body, have not consistently been shown to affect breast cancer rates, possibly because the levels of estrogen found in most of today's drug preparations are quite low. Advancing age is a risk factor that can also be partially explained by the effects of estrogen exposure: as a woman gets older, there is more time for her breasts to be exposed to the natural estrogen in her body. Almost 80% of breast cancers are diagnosed in women age 50 and older.

On the other hand, having a baby early in life and breastfeeding are thought to decrease a woman's exposure to cyclical estrogen because they suppress the menstrual cycle and, therefore, the risk of breast cancer is lowered. Moreover, some factors that increase a person's risk of breast cancer can be modified. Alcohol use, even only one drink per day, can increase a woman's risk of developing the disease. Obesity appears to increase risk, and some studies have shown that increasing one's activity level with a regimen of exercise can decrease the risk. It is unclear if the decreased cancer risk is due to weight loss or activity level, as these often go hand in hand. It may be that both the lost weight and the increase in activity are independently important. What seems to make sense is that a healthy lifestyle overall contributes to overall breast health.

Family history is another significant risk factor for developing breast cancer. Having a first degree relative (mother, sister or daughter) diagnosed with breast cancer, especially if they were diagnosed before the age of 40, almost doubles a woman's risk of being diagnosed with breast cancer during her lifetime. However, it is important to know that almost 80% of people diagnosed with breast cancer have no immediate family history of the disease.

It is estimated that almost 10% of breast cancers are caused by genetic mutations. Significant progress has been made in identifying genetic defects that are responsible for hereditary breast cancer syndromes. The most common genetic mutations occur in the genes known as *BRCA I* and *BRCA II*. Women who have a deleterious mutation in one of these two genes have a 50–80% chance of developing breast cancer in the course of their lifetime and have a higher risk of developing ovarian cancer. These genes account for a significant proportion, but not all, of inherited breast cancers. Other genes that have not yet been identified undoubtedly exist, and therefore a negative result from genetic testing, although reducing the likelihood of a genetic predisposition, does not entirely eliminate the possibility. A woman who has a significant family history of breast and ovarian cancer must still be followed closely.

Continued on page 48

The Nurse

Helen Carson

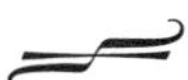

She was a nurse and proud of it!
Her license said so.
A cancer nurse, indeed.
Young and sweet
Swishy white uniform, squeaky shoes
With lofty goals

Making a difference.
Saving lives
Drying tears,
Hugging the pain.
So she thought,
Until that day

They told her she had it too.
Breast cancer, her doctor said.
She would have to have them both removed
Immediately; the day after her honeymoon!
She cried and railed, and retched with fear
And then she knew

She had never really made a difference.
How could she have?

She had not felt the rage and terror
The sleepless dreams of death and loss
Her future, her life, her legacy,
Or been so ill she wished to die,

Until the day the surgeon removed
The bandages and she looked down with tears
At the angry red gash where her breasts had been.
Breasts that had betrayed the woman within,
Subtle maybe, but seductive still,
And then she knew what her patients knew.

No one could make a difference.
No healer, no parent, no spouse, no friend.
The journey was made alone.
It was long...and cold...and dark.
But now when she met their eyes, they knew
She had finally become...the nurse.

Helen Carson was a registered oncology and hospice nurse for over 25 years. After three bouts of breast cancer, she left nursing and is now a training and technical assistance provider to Native American Head Start programs in California and Nevada. She recently received her master's degree in Educational Administration. She is a wife, a mom, a grandma, a friend, and an animal lover who enjoys reading and writing poetry, travel, cross stitching, photography, and flower gardening.

Part II
BREAKING THE NEWS

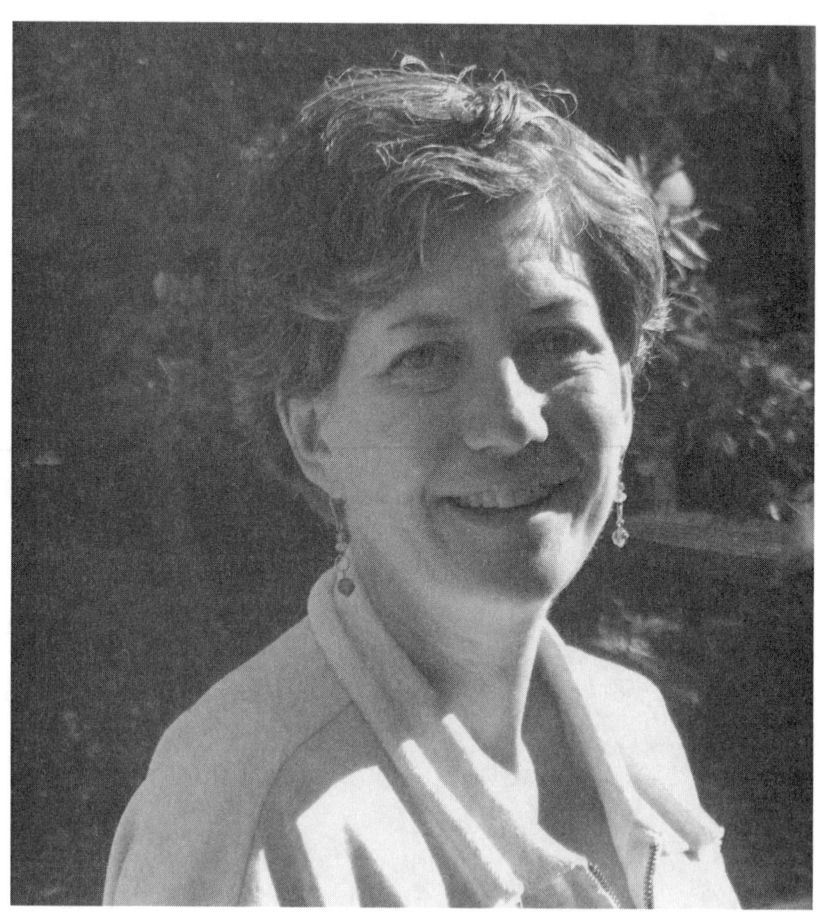

Jayne England Byrne

Throwing Down the Gauntlet

Jayne England Byrne

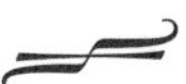

You have to make a lot of challenging decisions when you are diagnosed with breast cancer. Some of them are medical and some of them are philosophical. On the philosophical side, you have to choose a level of privacy. Who do you tell? When do you tell them? How much do you tell? It can be a very difficult choice, and it was for me. But I decided almost right away to throw down the gauntlet to the privacy challenge and be open about my disease and my struggles. I didn't want to be on this road alone. However, it is exhausting to revisit the same facts over and over. So I encouraged my inner circle to pass the word to extended family and mutual friends. I didn't care who knew that I had breast cancer as long as I didn't have to go through the repeated anguish of relaying the details.

About a month after my diagnosis though, I remained stumped about how to tell my far-flung friends about my cancer. How do you tell a friend from college, whom you haven't seen in over a decade and haven't talked to in two years? Do you say, "I've missed you. I have breast cancer. What's new on your end?" And I soon tired of everything being about me and my problem. I was hungry to listen to someone else's story.

My solution was to write a long letter: an actual snail mail letter on pretty paper. I wrote to childhood playmates I hadn't seen in years, college friends, former neighbors and a woman that I had worked with long ago. Altogether, I wrote to about twenty women in five different states. The beginning of the letter explained my cancer diagnosis and current medical condition. Then I asked them all for a favor. This was the close of my letter:

> *I count you among my friends, so I'll make the bold assumption that if we were talking you would say, "Jayne, is there anything I can do to help?" Well, in fact, you can.*
>
> *If you are the praying sort, your prayers are appreciated.*
>
> *And I have a request. Send me an email about YOU. The longer and more detailed the better! What are you up to? How are your kids, your parents, your job, your spouse, your boyfriend, your puppy, etc.? Do you have vacation plans? Are you remodeling your house? What have you been doing for fun lately?*
>
> *Nothing would make me happier than to open up my Inbox and find an email from you—about you. Truly, I am sick and tired of thinking about and talking about ME.*
>
> *Hope to hear from you soon!*
>
> *All my love,*
>
> *Jayne*

Every response was like a present. I expected replies, but I was taken aback by the beauty and the honesty that came to me. Sure, I heard about promotions and exciting vacations and all sorts of good news. But I also heard about troubled relationships, career obstacles and even (gasp!) children who were not quite perfect. Why did some of these women plunge into renewing an old friendship with no pretense? Perhaps it was because I had thrown down the gauntlet by opening myself up and letting them know that I was young, sick, scared and in need.

My story is still unfolding, as are the tales that were shared with me this past spring. While happy endings are not guaranteed, even a shred of hope can be amplified—for both the storyteller and the listener—once the truth is told.

Jayne England Byrne is a freelance writer and poet living in Greensboro, North Carolina. She was diagnosed with lobular breast cancer in March, 2006.

Continued from page 35

How Is Breast Cancer Detected?

Screening for breast cancer with *mammography*, unless one has a strong family history of breast cancer or a known genetic mutation that would require an earlier start, usually begins at age 40. Mammograms are intended to find cancers that are not detectable on physical exam, and ideally before they cause symptoms. The tumors detected by mammography are likely to be small, and the smaller the tumor is at the time of detection, the better the prognosis. However, most cancers are not found by screening studies. Because the most common presentation of a breast cancer is a painless new mass in the breast, breast self-exam and a clinical breast exam by a physician are important tools in detecting breast cancer at an early stage. Therefore, every woman should start breast self-exams in her 20's to get familiar with the way her breasts look and feel. Breasts are inherently lumpy and it is important for a woman to report any changes that are new or different and persist through a menstrual cycle. Aside from the presence of a new mass in the breast, other symptoms of breast cancer are swelling, skin changes, nipple inversion, nipple discharge or rash, or a lump under the arm.

If a *palpable* breast mass is detected, one that can be felt by hand, it needs to be pursued further. A mass must feel benign (noncancerous) on physical exam, look benign on radiological studies and appear benign pathologically to avoid surgery to remove it. Radiological studies may include a mammogram, *ultrasound*, and in selected cases, *magnetic resonance imaging* (MRI) or *ductogram*. Each of these technologies uses a different method to determine if a mass is benign or malignant-appearing. Mammograms use X-rays to look at the breast tissue. The level of radiation used is low and newer technologies such as *digital mammography* minimize the patient's exposure to radiation. Ultrasound, or sonogram, uses sound waves and can help distinguish a cyst, or a fluid-filled cavity in the breast, from a truly solid mass. If a person has dense breast tissue, ultrasound may visualize a mass that cannot be seen by mammography. Ultrasound will pick up a few of the cancers missed by mammogram, but if a mass is as dense as the breast tissue surrounding it, the mass will by undetectable by sonogram as well. MRIs use magnetic fields to create a picture of the mass and are probably the most sensitive test we have to detect a breast cancer. However, they are very expensive and time consuming and they sometimes find lesions that look suspicious but are really benign, which can lead to unnecessary biopsies and emotional distress. They need to be used with caution and in a very select group of women.

MRIs also do not detect 100% of breast cancers, and a benign-appearing MRI study does not always mean that cancer is absent. Even if a palpable mass appears benign using these techniques, a *biopsy*, the removal of cells or tissues for examination by a pathologist, still needs to be obtained. There are several kinds of biopsy procedures, including *fine needle aspiration* (FNA), *core biopsy*, *stereotactic biopsy*, or *surgical excision*. An FNA is the smallest and least invasive biopsy available. A thin needle is passed in and out of the breast mass and a collection of cells are pulled into the hub of the needle. These cells are then put on a slide and a pathologist looks at the sample under a microscope. When an adequate sample is obtained through this method, a trained *cytopathologist* can determine with 95% accuracy whether the mass is benign or malignant.

When a mass is large or is clearly seen on ultrasound, a *core biopsy* can be carried out. This type of biopsy requires local anesthesia and a small nick in the skin. A piece of the mass is removed through a large bore needle so that the tissue can be examined by the pathologist in its native configuration. If the lesion is only seen on mammogram, a similar biopsy, called a *stereotactic biopsy*, will be performed. With this test, the breast is placed in compression, as if a mammogram was being performed, and a needle is guided to the area in question with the aid of a computer. Samples of the mass are then extracted via the needle as the breast remains in compression. If a tissue diagnosis is not possible with the above methods or the findings from the pathology and the radiological studies are not in agreement, an *open surgical excision* is performed, removing the entire mass for further study.

Continued on page 72

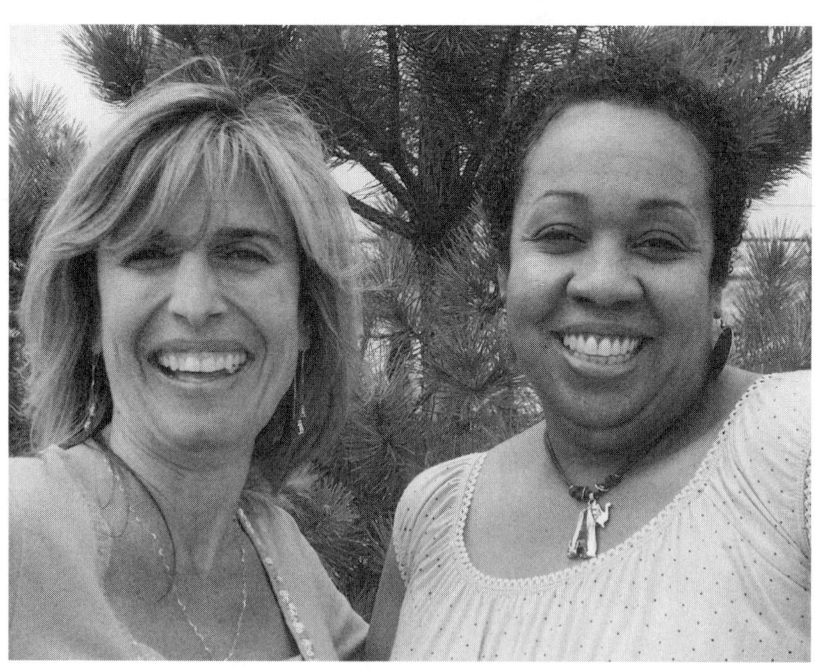

Erin Michele DiPaolo and Kim Larkin-Davis

Eat Your Chocolate Cake

Erin Michele DiPaolo

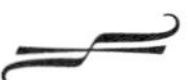

Kim, a fellow teacher at our school in Denver, had called a meeting. Last-minute meetings tend to make us all apprehensive. We sat, my co-workers and I, looking around the room at each other, wearing nervous smiles, waiting for it to begin. I bit my nails; others chatted. Would we be talking about wearing pajamas on Friday, as the first and second grade classes had earned pajama parties? Would we be discussing a shower for our principal, who had recently announced her wedding plans? A first grade teacher, Mrs. Hanson, announced that she had brought a chocolate cake to share. My mouth watered at the thought of it. Most women would agree that chocolate makes any occasion special, like a party. Mrs. Hanson dished up slivers of cake to most of the attendees. I requested a larger slice. I always do.

As we devoured the decadent cake, I noticed that Kim and her friend Mrs. Lindley held each other's hand. Good friends, I thought. What a blessing. Still, I wondered why they felt the need: it must be some huge announcement and it must not be good, I concluded.

Finally, Kim spoke to the group. She had had a mammogram over spring break, she said, and it had revealed a lump in her breast. She paused, trying not to cry, still squeezing Mrs. Lindley's hand ever so tightly. She'd had a number of biopsies and had been diagnosed with cancer. The group, normally so talkative, fell silent. This last-minute meeting had nothing to do with work. It had to do with how life can change in an instant.

Kim went on, saying that she didn't want anyone to change their behavior around her. In fact, she said, she had not wanted to make the announcement in the first place. She didn't want anything or anyone to change. She didn't want tears; no crying allowed; it was much too late for that. I looked around the room. There were no dry eyes. It was a powerful moment, one that defined what being a woman meant to me: being able to express grief so freely.

I also saw a community of people, educators, with different personalities and diverse views, bound together in their concern and empathy for this dear woman whom they all loved. Kim went on to say how truly blessed she felt to be able to work with such an incredible group of people. And then she broke down, but just a bit. It was a touching moment, and despite the terrible reason for it I found myself wishing for more meaningful moments when the souls of all of those around you are stirred. When she was asked if she needed anything, Kim simply said, "Lift me up in prayer." Some women in the room could relate to her request; others maybe not. But at that moment, I figured all would try. I did, and I have, every time I think of this courageous woman.

After the tears were wiped away, one teacher said, "Well, no one wants to eat their cake now." Kim ate, saying, "Eat your chocolate cake. Don't change what you do, who you are. Eat! That's what I'm going to do."

She asked that we not act differently because of her and here we were, already acting differently. Smart woman, Kim is. She knew human nature and that we are all so damned, well, human. We wanted to honor her request, really we did. But we could not change the fact that we were different now, changed by what she had said, transformed by her heartache and by the courage she had demonstrated. So I said I wanted mine even more. Not only because chocolate is a great comfort food, but also because life is short. You never know when it might be your last piece of chocolate cake. And so I ate.

I also thought of how this incredible woman was inviting us to live. She had cancer and she was urging, pleading with us to go on with life. Maybe our empathy was misplaced. She, after all, had won the fight already, regardless of the outcome. She had learned how to live above her circumstances. What a rare thing, a gift.

The meeting ended; each woman took her turn embracing Kim, speaking encouraging words to her. I waited patiently for my turn. I wanted to say everything in my heart. Mostly I wanted to give her hope and to let her know that if there was one thing I could do, it was pray.

And I also wanted to tell her something else. Nearly five years ago my mom was diagnosed with breast cancer. It was devastating to me, but not to my mom. She fought and she won. She didn't get sick once during chemotherapy; she didn't lose her hair, although she did lose a breast. She got the upper hand on death. I wanted Kim to know that she could, too. I wanted her to get a glimpse of what it looks like on the other side, after the surgery and drugs and everything else is over. The glory part.

We hugged. I told her I would pray; I told her my mom's story and I told her I loved her. In the end, isn't that all we really have? Love. I saw so much of it that Tuesday afternoon in a school in Denver, among friends, as we ate our chocolate cake.

A sports journalist with hundreds of stories published in *The Longmont Daily Times-Call*, the author is a freelance writer based in Colorado. A wife and mother whose passions include family, writing and travel, Erin has recently been published on *Colorado Magazine Online*, *Yourhub.com* and in *Read Five Magazine*.

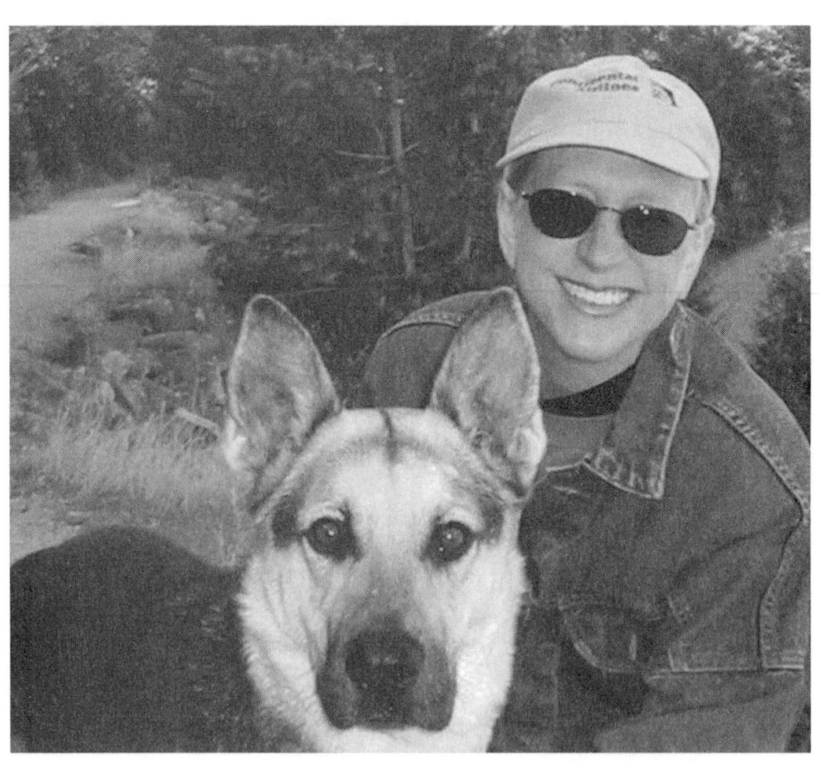

Barbara Plum Terrell

Are Ya Kidding Me?

Barbara Plum Terrell

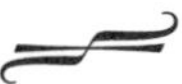

My case started with a routine mammogram and ended with black lace thong underwear.

At 43, I had my annual mammogram and the radiologist found something suspicious, a grouping of five microcalcifications. A microcalcification looks like a dot made by a large pencil. I had more mammograms and ultrasounds, followed by a stereotactic biopsy, which is like having a power screwdriver drilled into your breast, to remove suspicious tissue. I was then tagged, like Lassie. I'd been told that 90% of the time microcalcifications are not cancerous, so I wasn't worried about the test results.

I nearly passed out when the nurse called me at home the next afternoon. It was DCIS, *ductal carcinoma in situ*. Okay, I didn't pass out but I did stutter and ask her to repeat it about twenty times. How could I possibly have something I couldn't even spell?

I didn't cry when I gave my husband and parents the news. It wasn't until I was on the phone making an appointment with Julie at the surgeon's office that I suddenly found I couldn't talk and the tears flowed.

"Are ya kidding me?" was a phrase that I used over and over again during the next few months. At first, I racked my brain trying to figure out what I did to cause DCIS. Did I drink too much diet pop as a kid? (Chocolate Fudge was my favorite.) Was it because I grew up in the Midwest and was exposed to pesticides? No one knows why microcalcifications turn cancerous, so I'll never know why I was one of the chosen ones.

Next, I was faced with deciding my course of treatment. Lumpectomy? Mastectomy? Full or partial breast radiation? Sentinel node removal? It was like making a selection from a Chinese take-out menu. "Uh, yes, I'll have number 3, the lumpectomy and sentinel node removal with full breast radiation followed by tamoxifen, please."

What did I know about dealing with cancer? My family dies from heart attacks and strokes. I sat slumped on the sofa for a day trying to figure out how to handle it, when it hit me. I'd treat my cancer like a project at work. I sat up straight and grabbed a blank notebook. This just might work. From then on, my treatment was all business. I documented every conversation/phone contact/diagnosis/prognosis in my little black book. I magically felt much better because now I felt I had a plan of action.

I went back to work the following day, bringing with me two dozen of my favorite Lamar donuts. I wanted everyone to celebrate with me because I had the "good cancer" and since it was caught early, I was going to be OK. (I also figured it was harder to cry when you were stuffing your face with white fluff-filled, chocolate-covered Long Johns!) I also brought in my mammograms for an impromptu "show and tell" with my co-workers. I was the first one in the office to get cancer and my co-workers were speechless.

Frequent and effective progress reports are essential for a successful project. I started a "newsletter" to friends and co-workers via an email called *The Barb Report*. It was a wonderful way for me to let my friends know what was happening. The outpouring of positive thoughts and prayers that I received back was overwhelming. At times I felt like the luckiest person in the world.

Writing *The Barb Report* was very therapeutic. It allowed me to explain exactly what happened when I went through my biopsies (I had three of them), lumpectomies (I had two of those), and radiation treatments (twenty-five of those, but only on one breast). I explained the good, the bad, and the ugly. *The Barb Report* didn't pull any punches. I told everyone exactly what happened. I told everyone that the pain and recovery from the biopsies were worse than the lumpectomies. I told everyone about my pre-surgery routine. I had wires and tubes hanging out of my chest, and when the nurse said, "Come on honey, let's get another mammogram before surgery," I just about ran down the hall screaming. (That was definitely an "are ya kidding me" moment!) I told everyone what it was like to lie on a table for hours, naked from the waist up so the technicians could write on my chest with Sharpies to figure out where to put the tattoos for radiation treatments. I told everyone what it was like to go braless for months and that when I finally got to wear one again, there was more bra than me.

Several of my emails contained a section that I called "Lessons Learned." This was another take-off from the business world where, once a project is finished, you evaluate what went right and what went wrong. I want to share my findings on this project with you:

- When the doctor says, "You're going to feel a little pressure," he's really saying, "Your breast is going to be one humongous bruise tomorrow."
- I found out that if I had opted for a mastectomy, the insurance company would have been required to pay for a tummy-tuck to provide fat for breast implants. Hmm, free tummy-tuck and breast implants? There is a God!!
- The mammography machine was invented by a male physicist. I think he's now in the witness protection program.

- I'll probably need years of psychotherapy to get over having to massage my radioactive breast for an hour—a pre-surgery requirement so the doctor could find the "hot" lymph node—in a room with my dad and husband, as they talked about the stock market.

- The hardest part of the whole experience was not all of the needles or mammograms or ultrasounds or the MRI, but seeing tears in my father's eyes as I was wheeled away to surgery.

- When the doctor said, "A few patients experience the side effect of fluid gathering in one spot after the surgery," I assumed it wouldn't happen to me. Big mistake. Mine looked like a baseball growing out of my armpit. I named it Bernie and he hung around for several weeks.

- I now sport enough tattoos from radiation mapping to be an honorary biker chick.

- Insurance companies are evil. The latest snag is that my surgeon stopped accepting my insurance because she had to fight with them for every claim.

- Insurance companies are evil—I know, I said it before, but I have to say it again. To date, the insurance company has been billed a total of $55,000. They've paid out $22,000. Hmm, it makes my surgeon's decision to drop the insurance company understandable.

- Don't ever show your scars to relatives. I made this mistake over Christmas. I was feeling mighty smug that everything was finally starting to heal and, while still red, was looking pretty darn good. Well, I showed my chest and armpit to my mom and sister and now my mom thinks my ar pit is rotting and my sister thinks I have a connective tissue disease. Gee, and here I thought everything was looking great.

- I must be defective. My husband and I were stuck in a major traffic jam in the mountains for several hours. The only reading material in the car was a pamphlet on breast cancer. On the back cover was a lovely essay from a cancer survivor about how she used her cancer to "grow" and "mature", smell the roses, become a better person, etc. Me, I was mad as hell and didn't talk to God for weeks. I'm still in denial that it even happened. However, I did agree with the author that having cancer shows you just how much you are loved.

- Every time I have an ache, my mind automatically thinks, "Oh my God, has my cancer spread?" According to doctors and other survivors, this will be my automatic response to anything unusual for the next few years.

- The tests and surgery seemed very surreal and happened in such a short time that I never thought of myself as someone who had cancer. It really didn't hit me until I was at the radiation center and the nurse showed me the changing room. In it was a cubby hole for my changing gown with my name on it.

- The doctors, nurses and techs who worked with me should all be nominated for sainthood. They put up with my endless questions and were always smiling and laughing to make me feel better. (I hope it wasn't because I always wore my gown backwards!)

Well, it's been a little over six months since I was diagnosed. God and I are back on speaking terms. My mother's still in shock that I say words like "nipple" and "breast" in mixed company. I'm glad I was very open and vocal about my battle with breast cancer. Several of my friends have gotten mammograms for the very first time. Male friends have confided in me that they feel as if they are better equipped to handle breast cancer if their wives should be diagnosed.

How am I feeling? A few days before surgery, my husband and I walked and cried in the Susan B. Komen *Race for the Cure* in

Denver, with 65,000 others. Six days after having lumpectomies, I carried on a family tradition of hiking with my father about five miles at an altitude of 8,000 feet. I wasn't going to let a little thing like breast cancer get in the way. I also started to take belly dancing lessons because it's something I always wanted to do. I've never felt so loved by family, friends and co-workers, and now talk to my parents on the phone every day instead of twice a week. And finally, acupuncture has eliminated my tamoxifen-induced hot flashes. Yeah, I feel great!

And about the black lace thong underwear...when I went shopping to buy new bras that fit, the sales clerk said I just had to get the sexy matching lace thong underwear. I'd always thought thongs were worn on your feet. I couldn't even figure out the front from the back. Wait a minute, did she say sexy? I bought three pair!

Prompted to start writing nonfiction by her bout with breast cancer, Barbara's goal is to help others realize that they can make it through challenging times with humor. Previously published in *Voices of Lung Cancer: The Healing Companion*, Barbara lives outside of Denver where she and her computer guru husband share their home with a shy yet neurotic German Shepherd and a cat she calls "the evil one."

The Telling of It

Deborah Johnson

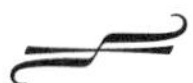

I froze in disbelief. At 51, after years of doing self-exams and finding nothing, I was standing in the shower on a December morning, water pouring over me, feeling this *thing* at the top of my left breast. I was dumbfounded and terrified. Eventually I stepped out of the shower, put on a bathrobe and, leaving a trail of damp footprints, slowly walked down the stairs of our Connecticut house.

Chip, my husband of nearly 30 years, was sitting at the dining room table reading the Sunday newspaper. "I don't want you to freak out," I said as I stood before him and opened my robe, "but tell me if this feels like something to you." With a slightly confused expression, he stood up and gently pressed where I was pointing. His eyes moved from my breast to my face. Not knowing what to say, we stared at each other and then hugged as tightly as we could. We stood like that for a long time before any words finally came out of me: "I'll call the doctor first thing tomorrow."

When you find a lump in your breast, all of a sudden those long waits for appointments disappear, and I was quickly booked with the gynecologist. "It could be a benign growth, a cyst," the doctor said, as he felt the little lump. "Let's get a mammogram and get you in to see a surgeon."

Then things really speeded up.

New Year's Eve was celebrated with a mammogram. The first week of the new year I saw the surgeon. After his examination, he got right to it: "There's a good potential that it is a malignancy," he said, and quickly began telling me of recent progress in the treatment of breast cancer.

He called two days later. Chip and I took the call together. The test was positive for cancer. I was not surprised—I was devastated. At that moment, all I could do was cry. Cancer! I wasn't thinking I could die, but that one dreaded word has such awful power. I laid my head in Chip's lap and sobbed as he stroked my hair. I could feel his body shaking, too. "Shhh," he said, running one hand over my hair as he held me tightly with the other. We sat like that for the rest of the evening, until I was too worn out from crying to do anything but sleep.

And then I was done with crying. Over the next couple of weeks, I went into action. I bought books and went on websites, searching for every bit of information that would prepare me for surgery, chemotherapy and whatever else was to come. I knew women who had had breast cancer, but I didn't call them. I wasn't ready to talk about it. Not until I had all the information, all the plans, all the details. I wanted to reach out to my family, but I felt this wasn't the time. And I absolutely dreaded telling my mother. My mother and I always had a strained relationship. I loved her, but she drove me crazy with her fault-finding and her impatience. Throughout my childhood and teenage years, I was the "good girl", doing exactly as she asked, wearing the clothes she liked (no jeans, no loafers), trying to please her and always afraid I would disappoint her. As I grew older, I learned how to handle her criticism better and overlooked her bad manners. I wasn't sure how she would handle this; our relationship was such that I had the ridiculous feeling I was letting her down.

The biopsy confirmed the previous test. Chip and I met with the surgeon for the details: Stage II cancer. Not the best case, not the worst.

I'd have to wait for more information from the biopsy lab tests to find out how bad things were. But we knew that surgery was required. The surgeon presented me with two choices: "breast-conserving" surgery that removes the tumor and the tissue surrounding it, or a modified radical mastectomy, taking the whole breast and some lymph nodes. He told me that the more limited surgery could mean another operation if cancer cells were found at the edges of the sample.

"What do you recommend?" I asked.

"I can only give you facts and options. It has to be your decision."

"What about survival rates?" I asked, not realizing then that this was probably the fourth time I had asked him the same question. His answer was the same each time: the cancer appeared small, caught early, and with treatment survival rates were very good.

My mind was in overdrive as we got in the car to go home.

"What do you think?" I asked Chip, as he drove us out of the parking lot.

"I think we should do what you believe is best." Ball back in my court. No one was going to decide for me.

"I think I should have the mastectomy," I said. "I want them to take it all. I don't want to have to go back for a second surgery."

"I agree," Chip said, taking his eyes off the road to look at me. "Are you okay with that?"

"If someone's going to be cutting into my body," I answered, "it's not going to be more than once, not if I can help it!" Wow! When I said the words, I felt as though a burden had been lifted. But another remained: while I never doubted my husband's love and devotion, I would be disfigured by the mastectomy. "But I'm going to have one breast," I said.

"But I'll still have *you*. And don't forget," he said with a smile, "I've always been a leg man."

The surgery was scheduled for Friday, February 19th. Now I could tell people. In what I could only construe as comic timing, on the day before the biopsy I had been promoted to News Director at the Connecticut television station where I had worked for fourteen years. Running a television newsroom is a pressure-filled job but it would keep me busy and leave me little time to brood. I began by telling my managers and staff, first individually, then in small groups and finally in the larger arena of our morning staff meeting. I wasn't uncomfortable: we had worked together for so long and on so many tragic stories and events. Here was another crisis, although an extremely personal one. So I had no problem standing up and saying, "I have breast cancer." Then I contacted some friends scattered around the country, all of whom were supportive.

This left my family to tell. It would be very hard to tell my two sisters that I had a killer disease. I called Stephanie, my youngest sister, first. She lived across the country, near San Diego. She cried. And cried and cried. "Do you want me to come out there?" she asked between sobs. "No," I said. "There's nothing to do. What would we do, sit and look at each other all day and cry?" I told her to try to think positive thoughts. And to say nothing to our mother. My middle sister, Marian, had the same reaction: tears and fears. "Think positive thoughts," I asked. "And don't tell Mommy."

That was it: my mother was the only person left to tell. And it had to be face-to-face.

Two weeks before the surgery, Chip and I drove to my mother's house in New York, on Long Island's North Shore. A cold, clear afternoon, just a few days past my 52nd birthday. She expected our visit, something we did every couple of months. I left the car and walked up the flagstone path to the door, filled with apprehension about the task at hand.

I knocked, opened the door, stepped in. "Hello, we're here!" I called out. I heard the TV, the volume high because her hearing was bad and she refused to wear a hearing aid. We walked towards the sound. Perched on the edge of the loveseat in the den, the TV remote in her hand, Mom looked up. "Hi there," she said. She was wearing a floral cotton housedress over slacks. Chip gave her a kiss, "Hi, Nettie," he said, and sat in the nearby armchair. I sat next to her and kissed her cheek.

She did not look good and hadn't for a long time. I studied her while she gazed at the TV. She looked all of her 81 years. Age, high blood pressure and emphysema had taken their toll on her. Her face was mottled; the skin puffy. Her breathing was labored. Her arms were covered in bruises, her thin skin and her medications conspiring to show off every bang and bump.

I told her I had something she needed to know. Click. The TV went black. She turned to me.

"Mom, I have breast cancer."

Her eyes first grew wide then pinched shut. I waited what seemed like an eternity, praying that my news wouldn't provoke her usual anger, criticism or words of blame. Then her face crumpled and she started to wail.

"Oh no, oh no. No, no."

"The surgery is in two weeks," I said, not sure if she was listening. Her arms wrapped tightly around her chest, she began to rock back and forth, still wailing. "No, no, no. Why, why?" she cried. "We don't have it in our family."

"Mom, it's just bad luck. It happens. But the doctors say the prognosis is good, that we caught it early and the treatments these days are very effective." I didn't think she heard me. Rocking and wailing, rocking and wailing. Then she said something that startled me, that brought tears flooding to my eyes: "Oh, why couldn't it be me?" she cried. "Why can't it be me?"

She repeated it like a mantra, over and over. My heart stopped. The woman who had found fault in everything I'd done, or so I thought, wanted to take on my cancer, take it away from me!

I wrapped my arms around her heaving shoulders and put my head against hers. We rocked and cried together. All of my problems with my mother disappeared in that instant. Instead, I held on to my mother, one of the only constants in my life. Even though I was the one with the cancer, at that moment she needed the consolation. And I was so very happy to give it.

A native of Long Island, New York, Deborah enjoyed a successful career in local television, producing public affairs and news programs and as News Director at *WFSB-TV* in Hartford, Connecticut. Now eight years cancer free, Deborah is enjoying life with her husband Chip in San Diego, California.

Part III

I'VE CHANGED

Shedding Hair

Diane Payne

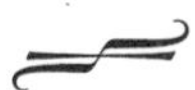

"Is the water too hot?" I ask Mom as she leans her head under the kitchen sink faucet.

"No, it's perfect," she answers.

Wearing only a stained polyester bathrobe and worn-out slippers, Mom smiles as if she is a queen being waited on hand and foot.

"Doesn't it feel good when the water trickles down your neck?"

"Yeah. You're as good as the girls at Ottie's shop. When you grow up, you'll be a good beautician."

"You mean that, Ma?"

"Wait until you get older, you'll see. Some of the girls burn your scalp. Don't even check the water before sticking your head under. You won't be lazy like them. You got to let your nails grow though. That's what the women like. A nail massage."

While Mom talks, the sink fills with her hair. I say nothing, hoping the hair will quit falling out. Dad warned us that Mom might lose her hair now that she has started chemotherapy treatments, but I didn't think it'd be like this. I don't know what to do. I'm afraid it will all fall out if I keep scrubbing, or that the force of the water will make her hair peel away like dead leaves shaking off a tree on a windy day. I don't know how I'll wrap what little hair is left in the pink spongy curlers next to me on the counter. Mom keeps talking about her hairdressers as if she has enough hair to return there next Friday.

I towel dry what's left as if nothing has happened, hoping she won't turn her head and look at the sink, which is now filled with blackish gray hair. First she loses her breast and now her hair. And she's only thirty-three years old. That seems old to me but not old enough to be dying and losing parts of your body. As I pat Mom's hair dry, I try to say how clean her scalp smells but the tears begin to build and the words choke up inside me.

"What's wrong?"

"Nothing, Ma. Nothing."

"Thought you were crying there for a minute," she says, while I hold the towel tightly over her head, praying that when I remove it, God will have grown her a new batch of hair. When I take off the towel, I expect a miracle. Instead, there is more hair clinging to the towel. I blame myself for every hair that falls out. If I hadn't washed her hair, it would still be there. Then I remember the hair on her pillowcase and blame God. God is supposed to be a miracle worker but I don't know who he saves those miracles for.

I pick up a curler and try to wrap the remaining hair. I slowly work the hair around the sponge and snap the curler in place, praying that the hair will quit falling out.

"You don't have to wrap it too tight," Mom says.

"I won't, Ma. Does this feel all right?"

"Perfect."

It's working better than I expected. Six curlers are in and she doesn't look too bald with the hair wet and bunched up in curlers. I put a few more in and wonder how I'll be able to keep her away from the mirror. She always looks before I finish setting it and she'll notice the missing hair. I wanted to make her feel good, feel queenly, but it's not going to work out that way.

"Can you tell that I'm losing any hair?"

This question takes me by surprise. She has never talked about it before. "Yeah, but it's not too bad."

"Not yet," she says. "Just about everyone going to therapy is bald. But it grows back. They say it'll grow back thicker than before."

"How long does it take for the hair to fall out?"

"Some say it fell out the very next day after the first treatment. Others don't even lose all of it, just some. Maybe I'll be one of the lucky ones."

"I hope so, Ma."

As I wrap the next curler, I remember my long hair and how good it felt when Mom brushed it. Last year the barber cut my hair off. Mom's arms had swollen from her cancer and my hair was becoming a nuisance; Dad thought I was selfish, asking Mom to brush it before bed. Mom moaned when she wrapped my hair into a tight bun and I moaned because my skin was stretched too tight. But at least she touched me when I had hair. I had hoped she would try to stop me from cutting it, but she didn't. I came home with a pixie haircut and Mom said she liked it. I wanted her to cry as I did, riding my bike home from the barbershop, but she didn't. She took the bag of my hair and put it in her bottom dresser drawer with all the other special things she saved. No longer did she brush my hair at night, running her fingers over my scalp, with each stroke whispering a secret "I love you" message. Now my hair was short and convenient.

"You ever miss your long hair?"

Her question frightens me. I'm sure she's reading my mind. "Not really, Ma." I lie but maybe she won't catch this one.

"Hair isn't that important, is it? We're lucky we have eyes. I'd hate to be blind. We got a lot to be thankful for, don't we?"

"Yeah, I'd hate to be blind. Or have polio like Karen."

"We are lucky, aren't we?"

"Yeah, Ma."

After I wrap the last curler, Mom runs her fingers through her hair, checking the tightness of the curlers. "Let me see the mirror."

It's the kind with two sides: one side a regular mirror and the other a magnifier. First she looks through the magnifier side, then the regular, then back through the magnifier. Then she looks at me. I remain quiet. She looks at the floor and sees all the hair that has fallen. She cries, forgetting the blindness and polio, seeing only baldness.

"Ma, I'm going to let my hair grow back long, longer than before. I'm going to make a wig for you."

She cries, and says nothing.

"Ma, you're still beautiful. You got to believe that. I still love you, no matter what. There's still some hair left. Yours will grow back thick, remember? Soon it'll be the length of mine. Ma, it ain't forever. Stop crying, please. It's just hair."

We both know there will be none left when the hair dries and the curlers are pulled out. Her hair will unravel from the curlers and fall to the ground, joining the rest. Mom is thinking about beauty, yet I know that having hair is about being touched: she will miss the trips to the beauty shop, her sisters dyeing it, and even my washing and setting it. Suddenly my short hair feels long and I know I'll let it grow to make that wig.

Diane Payne lives with her teenage daughter in a small town in Arkansas where she teaches creative writing at the local university. She has been published in hundreds of magazines and is the author of the memoir *Burning Tulips*.

Continued from page 47

Understanding the Pathology Report

We have already seen that a tumor found in the breast may be benign or malignant. We also discussed the differences between lobular carcinoma and ductal carcinoma, and what makes a cancer invasive or pre-invasive. Equally important in determining the future course of the disease is knowing the *grade* of the tumor. The grade of the tumor tells us the tumor's potential for growth. Tumor grade is determined by examining the appearance of various structures within the tumor, such as the cell nuclei, and the rate of cell division. A *low grade* or *well differentiated* tumor is slower growing and approximates normal tissue; a *high grade* or *poorly differentiated* tumor is fast growing and the cells are very abnormal-looking; an *intermediate* or *moderately differentiated* tumor is in the middle.

Another important component of evaluating a cancer is to determine if the tumor is *estrogen receptor* (ER) or *progesterone receptor* (PR) positive or negative. A normal breast cell has receptors on its surface that allow estrogen and progesterone to attach to the cell, stimulating it to grow. If a tumor cell has the same receptors, it will also grow and divide more rapidly in the presence of estrogen or progesterone. These tumors can be treated with medications that block the receptors or lower the levels of the hormones in your body, often in combination with chemotherapy, slowing the tumor's growth.

HER2 is a gene that helps control cell growth by increasing the production of a cell surface protein. If there are too many copies of the gene present, the cell receives signals to grow and multiply. These tumors are thought to be more aggressive than tumors that are HER2 negative. However, there are newer drugs that can target cells that are HER2 positive, slowing their growth, and these drugs have been shown to be very effective in improving survival.

Once breast cancer is diagnosed, the disease needs to be *staged* in order to determine the treatment needed and the prognosis a patient faces. The stage is based on tumor size, whether the cancer has spread to the lymph nodes under the arm, and whether the disease has spread to parts of the body beyond the breast and lymph nodes. Ductal carcinoma in situ is *Stage 0* disease: the cancer cells are contained within the duct and have not spread into the surrounding tissue. The disease cannot spread to other parts of the body and the long-term survival is 99%. *Stage I* disease is a tumor smaller than two centimeters that has not spread to the lymph nodes under the arm. *Stage II* disease is one where the tumor is 2 to 5 centimeters in size and the cancer has spread to up to three lymph nodes. It also includes tumors greater than 5 centimeters in size without nodal involvement. *Stage III* tumors are less than or equal to 5 centimeters with four or more positive nodes or larger than 5 centimeters with any nodal involvement. *Stage IV* disease refers to patients who have disease outside of the breast and in the nodes found under the arm.

Continued on page 90

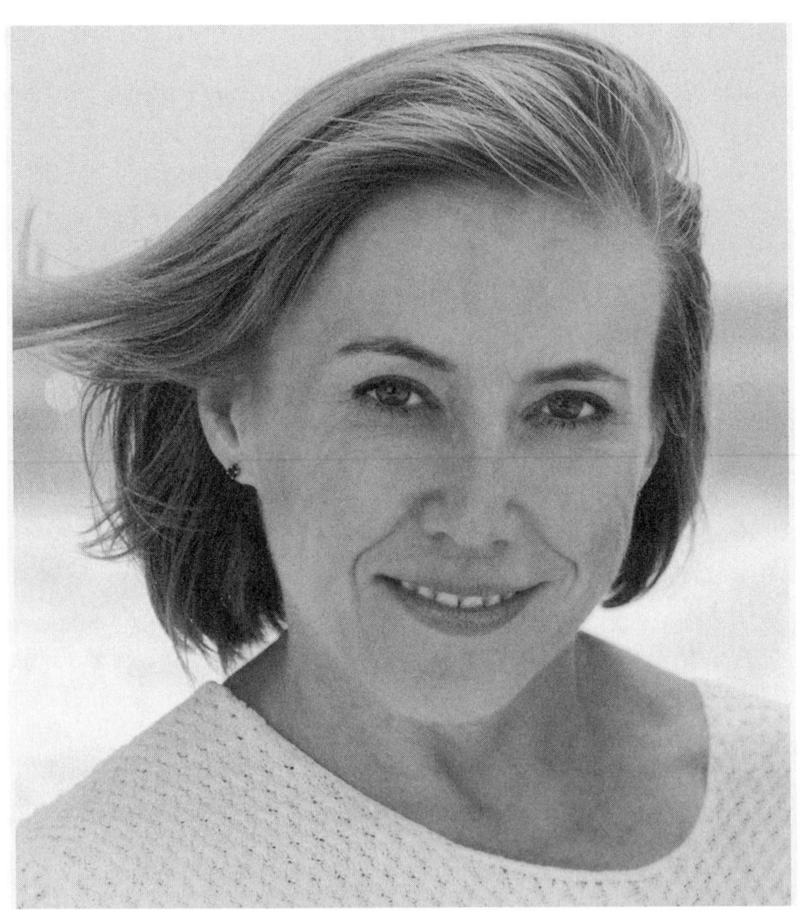

Virginia Hardee Silverman

Sister

Virginia Hardee Silverman

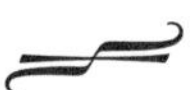

Anyone who saw us sitting in the bar might have assumed we were on a date that was going very badly. While Emily cried, I held her hand, not saying a word, listening to her tear-choked words of fear and desperation. From time to time, I touched her hair, pushing it away from the edge of her face, giving her sobs full freedom to pull and push. Rod Stewart blared over the lounge speakers, begging her to cry harder and louder. The table was littered with Kleenex, a white sea of spent feeling.

My lunch date's wispy blond hair parted across her small neck as she bent her head to hide her tears. Emily had been diagnosed with breast cancer the week before. She was now trying to decide whether to amputate both of her breasts, eliminating the possibility of recurrence. The alternative was to hang on to the so-far-unaffected left breast and just deal with the afflicted side. Either option represented a huge loss. I could feel every inch of her anger at life and God for doing this to her. I had faced the same decision four years earlier. I chose to go for broke and surrendered both my breasts. Recurrence aside, symmetry proved to be important to me as well.

"I just can't believe this is happening to me. I don't want to be cut up. I don't want to die, but I don't want the scars. I love my breasts just like they are. I've always been told that my breasts are my best feature. How will I ever be comfortable being undressed in front of anyone again?"

Emily had not yet been married, had no children and no immediate prospects for either. She saw her diagnosis as a life sentence of loneliness. She was sure that no one would want her without her breasts. All I could do was try to listen to her and try not to remember my own fear of the future. If we were both in trauma, I was sure we'd never make it out of the restaurant.

I held off memories of my own panic and tried to reassure her. "I know you feel this way now, but you have to remember the most important thing is to save your life. You want to live. That's all that matters. You want to avoid having to go through this again, so giving up the other breast will prevent you from having to face this horrible decision again." It would also reduce her cancer's forty percent chance of recurrence to almost nothing. She had already had two lumpectomies and radiation on the breast that was the site of the recurrence. If she chose the most aggressive course of treatment, this would be her last.

My own words sounded hollow to me as I remembered my own fright four years ago. I had no one then to help me through the process. I remembered sitting alone at my computer searching for information and direction. The only person I knew with breast cancer, Sally, had died three months before my diagnosis, after an eight-year battle with the disease. I saw her whittle away to almost nothing, the result of a mastectomy, two bone marrow transplants, five rounds of chemo, and two brain surgeries. She had been my trailblazer, leaving crumbs along the way for me to follow when my time came. But even with the memory of her wise personal choices to light my way, I felt blind and overwhelmed. I needed someone living who could promise life after the knife. I made a promise to myself to reach out whenever I could to help other women who faced these decisions.

I told Emily that I chose to start reconstruction during surgery, so that when I woke up I would have some shape. I just didn't want to come to and feel concave. The implants I have feel natural. "They even bounce when I jog," I quipped. She laughed a little then. Her tear-filled eyes brightened for a second, perhaps filled with a vision of a normal future filled with exercise and luncheons and shopping sprees.

"When you walked in here," she said, "I never would have guessed that you had a double mastectomy. You look great." Yes, I was now the proud owner of two Inamed 153 silicone implants, 350cc's each, which represented an increase of one whole cup over my natural breasts' size. She smiled again. A little smile. Her breath was calmer and stronger now. Her eyes, although red-rimmed and edged with fear, were clearer. Suddenly, I had an idea.

"Do you want to see them? My breasts, I mean. If you're interested, we could go into the ladies room and I could show you what the scars look like after four years. Hell, you can even touch them if you want to." We started giggling like two schoolgirls about to share a really juicy secret. "Check please," Emily said loudly, and we both laughed.

We left our cocktails on the table and moved with determination toward the ladies room. Once inside, we went directly to the handicapped stall; it seemed appropriate under the circumstances. Emily stared as I unbuttoned my blouse, eager to catch a glimpse of what she would look like on the other side of the surgery.

I had never deliberately shown my breasts to another woman before. I found it strangely exhilarating, seeing the look of child-like anticipation on Emily's face. I opened my blouse to reveal my 36Cs. "The scars are almost gone," I pointed out. "You can only see them if you look closely." Emily leaned in, trying to find the re-sewn skin. "Wow, they look fantastic," she said. Almost with envy. Almost with admiration. I was proud to show her my bulging badges of courage.

I arched my back. "Go ahead. You can touch them if you want. I won't feel it. One of the things that happen from the surgery is that you lose all the nerves in the front of your breasts." She reached out with one finger and pressed on the side of my left implant. "God, they feel so natural," Emily gasped. "I can't believe it."

"That's what good silicone will do for you," I answered. Emily's panic was subsiding. I could tell she could picture herself with my breasts, or her version of my breasts. I could tell she could see herself living beyond the surgery.

"So, what are you going to do?" I asked as I buttoned up. "Are you going to go for it?"

She paused a moment. Her eyes dropped back to my chest and rose finally to meet my gaze. "Yeah, I think I can do this. I want to live, and I don't want to have to go through this again." I understood exactly how she felt.

"How about we finish our drinks and talk about your new cup size? Some days I wish I had gone for Ds." I put my arm around her shoulders and coached her back into the crowded room.

Born and raised in rural eastern North Carolina, the daughter of a sometime tobacco farmer, Virginia Hardee Silverman spent her childhood playing on the wooded banks of the Tar River. She has been a marketing executive with Fortune 50 companies for 24 years and recently completed her Master of Fine Arts degree in Creative Non-Fiction at Antioch University in Los Angeles. Her first manuscript, *The Virginia Monologues*, is a collection of personal essays about her life. She has been breast cancer free for five years and is passionate about helping others who find themselves facing this daunting disease.

Hair Alone

Phyllis S. Hillinger

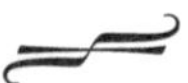

Standing in the checkout line at the supermarket, I smile at the smartly dressed woman in front of me. I haven't seen her in years and I strain to pull her name from the spidery web of my memory. She returns my smile, but it's obvious she doesn't have a clue who I am. I tell her my name, and she says, "Oh, you look so different with your short hair." And I do.

Over the last year, I have had this experience many times; I can hide in plain sight. This phenomenon is both unsettling and freeing at the same time. I smile at folks on my way around town, the place where I've lived for thirty years, and people present their pleasant faces without a sign of knowing me. My errands are efficient, not interrupted by the kind of chatty conversations that happen when a person runs into someone at the post office or drug store. I'm spared the time-wasting discussion of the weather and of what my grown children are doing and where they are living now. They don't hear about my work, travels, or aches and pains, and I don't hear about theirs.

I move through town as an anonymous citizen. My anonymity means I don't have to repeat again for those not in my close circle that a routine mammogram revealed shadows that turned out to be cancer. I don't have to say that I was strong going into 16 weeks of chemotherapy and I'm strong coming back to long walks, weights at the gym, and, finally, writing. I can skip telling them that I didn't need a "wake-up" call; I've been married to a physician for 37 years. I know illness can cancel both work and play and I don't take the ordinary tasks of life for granted. I can bypass these philosophical details because my hair is short and nobody knows me.

My family and close friends say I look younger, more artsy, a little alternative—all pleasing adjectives. Who wouldn't want a fresh new look at 58? But I haven't deliberately made this hairstyle choice. Though my hairstylist urged me to crop it years ago, my new youthful "do" is a by-product of chemotherapy, a fact that I can't dismiss lightly. I still have the auburn wig I wore for the summer when my head was bald, before I grew this inch of my own. During the time when I wore the wig, I would pass a mirror and wonder who that stranger was peering back at me. At a meeting with writing pals, I tearfully admitted that I didn't know who I was any more. I couldn't muster the energy to write and I couldn't research the scary topic of breast cancer. I just wanted to live through the "magic drugs" that would hopefully destroy the cancer cells, and I wanted my old healthy self back.

Now I'm beginning to feel like the old me and I'm getting used to my new image. I like wash-and-wear hair that requires nothing more than a little mousse and a random scrunch to style. I like seeing my earrings dangle free. But now I also find myself looking at women with short hair and wondering if their hairstyle is one they chose because it's easy to care for, or fashionable—or because they're waiting for hair follicles to spring back to life. I smile at those women who seem to be looking at me with the same questioning gaze, and I nod my head as if to say, "I know what you endured. You look different with your short hair, but I recognize you."

After a career writing for not-for-profit organizations, at 50 Phyllis Hillinger began writing personal essays, short stories and poetry, often on the subject of her life growing up on the Massachusetts shore. She and her husband Stephen, an oncologist, have raised two sons and two daughters and now enjoy traveling, sailing, long walks in the Adirondacks and Stephen's Belgian waffles, reported to be the best in the world.

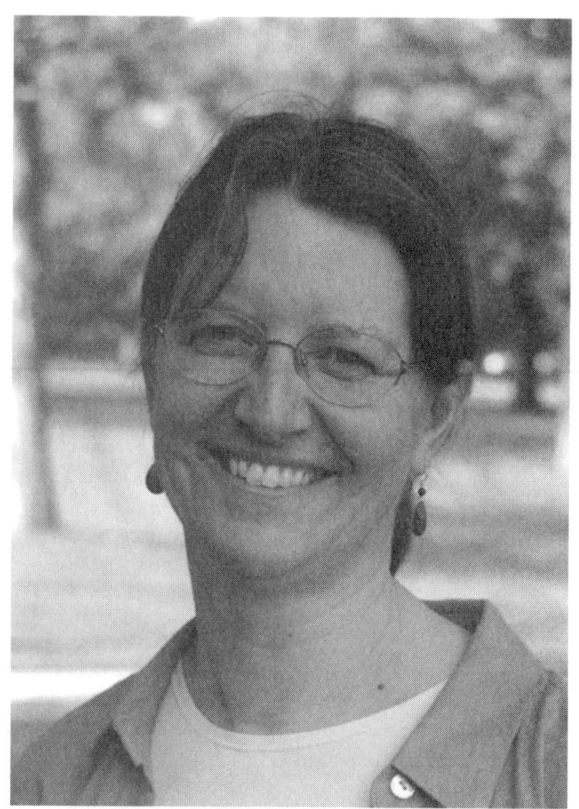

Kathleen Henderson Staudt

God's Wounds

Kathleen Henderson Staudt

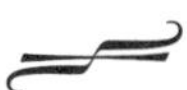

For a Christian and a writer who has recovered from breast cancer, the opportunity presents itself to explore some pretty heavy metaphysical connections and ironies. I have found that sometimes these connections between sacred and secular experiences can be illuminating, as if the Holy Spirit were saying of the Gospels, "Pay attention: the two modes of experience are connected. You were given these stories for a reason." So here goes...

The thing about surgery for breast cancer is that it changes you forever. Of course, we make a great effort, during the recovery process, to assure ourselves and the world around us that we are OK after all. The lumpectomy wound heals; we have reconstructive surgery or buy "natural looking" prostheses that feel real to the touch. We do our best to look the same and feel the same, on the outside.

But for me, it never felt exactly the same on the *inside*. This is now a different body, even though it is my own; it is a new thing. I have gotten used to it, just as I have adjusted to the irrevocable changes that came after a pregnancy, or that come now with aging.

The transformation happened awfully fast. I was only 37. I had two small children. Less than a month passed between the first "suspicious" mammogram and the mastectomy. So it took some getting used to. Since I chose not to have reconstructive surgery, there is an empty space on that side, and a scar. It took some time for me to get to the point where I could look at myself in the mirror and say "this is how I look now" and not burst into tears, but I finally did. And I cannot really escape thinking about what might have been if it hadn't been caught early. The suddenness of the discovery and the drastic nature of the cure have left me with a much deeper and immediate understanding of the tenuousness of life and health.

By the grace of God, I have been able to recover and go on with my life. I see the years that followed as a "new life"—illuminated and made more precious by this experience of serious illness. But I do not want to deny what has happened to me, even if I could: the evidence is right there, carved on my body, for the rest of my life.

Christians believe that the Risen Lord still bore on His hands and His side the wounds inflicted at the Crucifixion. Those wounds did not disappear when He rose from the dead. Indeed, for the apostle Thomas, those wounds were the evidence that the Lord showed to prove that He is who He is: potent reminders that resurrection, transformation, and newness of life come at a price. The price is not forgotten, but redeemed and glorified in the victory of new life. The wounds on that resurrected body do not deny, but affirm a passage through genuine and truly awful human suffering and death.

Most of us don't dwell on it much and I have enough generations of insistently Protestant blood in me to shrink from attention to such a baroque subject as "God's wounds" (so sacred a subject, in fact, that it was considered an oath in Shakespearean English). But we were given this story for a reason.

And so, sometimes, when I catch a glimpse of myself in the mirror, dressing in the morning, and see that scar and that empty place, I remember the encounter with my own mortality and I rejoice in the life that has been given back to me. Perhaps I would have the same feeling of relief and deliverance recovering from some other ailment. But the thing about breast cancer and the operation called a "total simple mastectomy" is that it is very incarnational: the evidence of the operation which has saved, and changed, my life is right there, spelled out for me on my own flesh. It's like getting a quick and inescapable review of the Gospels' central message, any morning I choose to consider it in front of the mirror. The Spirit gives odd gifts sometimes, and for me, this has been a gift indeed.

Dr. Kathleen Henderson Staudt works as a teacher, poet and spiritual director at a number of institutions in the Washington, D.C. area, including the Virginia Theological Seminary and the University of Maryland. Her poetry, essays and reviews have appeared in *Christianity and Literature*, *Cross Currents*, *Sewanee Theological Review*, *Living Prayer*, *The Anglican Theological Review*, and *Weavings*, among others. She is the author of *At the Turn of a Civilization: David Jones and Modern Poetics*, published in 1994, and *Annunciations: Poems out of Scripture*, published in 2003. Information on her other work exploring the breast cancer experience can be found at www. poetproph.blogspot.org.

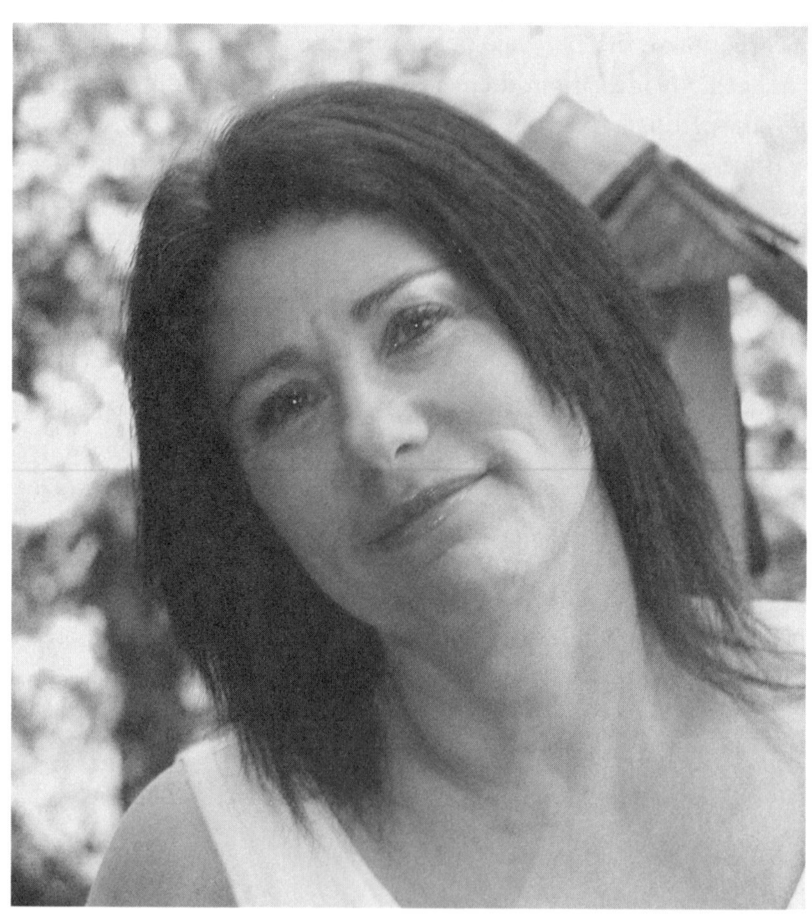

Marcie Beyatte

Losing My Hair

Marcie Beyatte

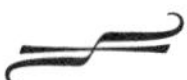

When I was very young, I would go to the beauty parlor with my grandmother and watch while she had her hair marcelled into soft waves. I'd collect abandoned scraps of hair from the floor and sort them into piles by color and then by shade. My own curly hair didn't belong to me yet: my mother was in charge and she would roughly wash, comb, and try to tame my curls with barrettes. It was always tearful work. As a teenager, my best friend and I scorched each other's hair as we ironed out our curls between towels, but nothing worked. In time, I came to accept my curly-headed reality. But well into adulthood, three years ago, I had my hair professionally straightened at a downtown salon. For the first time in my life, I loved my hair. It was shiny and smooth and I could toss it. For two weeks, I enjoyed blowing it dry and using new hair products.

Then a routine mammogram diagnosed breast cancer and I learned I'd have to go through chemo and lose my hair. That I would also lose a breast seemed less traumatic at the time. For the six weeks before treatment started I had a love affair with my dark, shoulder-length hair, made sweeter knowing that we were soon to part.

I was told I would begin losing my hair after the first treatment. I didn't want to lose it handful by handful, but I didn't want to shave my head alone. So I planned a formal shaving party, for a date after my first round of chemo, and invited my friends to witness the event. I bought a wig to wear after the deed was done and insisted that my friends wear wigs or hats for the occasion.

The day of the party approached and my hair had not yet begun to fall out. Did I have the courage to shave my head *before* it started leaving on its own accord? At spin class three days before the party, I wiped sweat from the back of my neck and a big wad of hair stuck to my palm. I was relieved in a sense; the party could go on as planned.

On the afternoon of my head-shaving party, my sister braided my hair into ten braids so I could donate it to *Locks for Love*, an organization that uses human hair to make wigs for kids undergoing chemo. My friends gathered in the garden wearing a hilarious assortment of wigs and hats. The wine flowed. After we were all sufficiently warmed up, I seated myself in a chair placed in the middle of the outdoor deck and draped a towel, barber-style, around me. My son began, cutting off my braids, and then my husband took over with the buzzer. The scissors hurt because the blades were dull and the sound of the buzzer was deafening. But soon all that remained of my hair was a heap on the deck, already beginning to waft away in the breeze. That I didn't harbor any disfiguring scars or carbuncles on my scalp was a relief; my friends commented on my beautifully shaped head. I took a quick shower and made an entrance in my wig and a long caftan, like an old-fashioned starlet.

After the party I dutifully wore my wig when I greeted the mailman and wore a kerchief at the gym. After two weeks of this, I realized I was hiding my baldness as if I were ashamed. In spin class, riding beside my bald friend Zane, I ripped off my babushka, thinking that if he could be bald, so could I. I no longer felt like a badly made-up drag queen.

The hardest test was going grocery shopping bald. The first time I made the attempt, I had my wig beside me in the car. I cried as I chickened out and donned it at the last minute. The next time I succeeded, but I was convinced everyone was staring at me. After about ten or twenty times I forgot to notice and after about fifty or sixty times I forgot to care.

I was bald for weeks and weeks after treatment ended. After three months, my hair looked like the gray lamb coat my Russian grandmother used to wear. After six, I had steel gray curls that lay close to my skull. After a year, I had a serious Afro in which I could hide small objects. After eighteen months, close friends told me that I might consider wearing a hat. All the time.

It was time to make a decision; either I'd cut my hair into a more human shape or get it straightened once more. I chose to straighten it, and regained a smooth cap of hair covering my ears. My hair could once again blow in the wind. I felt like me again.

A cancer survivor since 2003, Marcie Beyatte found that after treatment she could no longer say, "One day I will." She learned to say, "Today I am." She is the creator and producer of the program *Cancer in So Many Words*, the mission of which is to encourage cancer survivors to express themselves through writing. Marcie's essays have appeared in the *Contra Costa Times* and *The Monthly.* Marcie received the 2006 Leap of Faith Award and she was a delegate at the LIVESTRONG Survivors Summit in Austin in October 2006.

Continued from page 73

Treating Breast Cancer

There are many treatment options for patients with breast cancer. These include *surgery*, *chemotherapy*, *radiation*, *endocrine therapy* and *immunotherapy*. These therapies are defined as either *local* or *systemic* treatment. Local therapies (surgery and radiation) treat the breast and *axillary* (underarm) region. Chemotherapy, endocrine therapy and immunotherapy treat cells that may have left the breast and traveled to other parts of the body.

Most women with breast cancer will need some type of surgery. Surgery is used to remove the tumor, check to see if disease has spread to the lymph nodes under the arm, and, in cases of advanced disease, remove bulky tumors to relieve discomfort. There are two main choices for surgery in the breast. One is a *mastectomy*, the removal of the entire breast, which may be performed with or without reconstruction of the breast. The other is a *wide excision* (sometimes referred to as lumpectomy), the removal of the tumor along with a wide margin of normal tissue around the tumor, followed by radiation. Radiation is treatment with high energy X-rays to shrink or kill any tumor cells that may be left behind but cannot be seen. Radiation is usually delivered as a beam of energy from a large machine. The patient lies on the table for approximately 5 minutes in the same position while the radiation is delivered to the affected area. This form of radiation is delivered five days a week for just over 6 weeks in most cases. *Internal radiation* involves administering radiation through tubes or a balloon placed in the breast. The advantage to this regimen is that it takes a much shorter period of time to complete, usually only one week. Recent studies have also shown that in some women with aggressive forms of breast cancer, radiation may be used even in the case of a mastectomy, so one cannot assume that having a mastectomy will allow the patient to avoid the need for radiation.

More and more women are opting to keep their breast if it's possible to do so with an acceptable outcome. This decision, along with the definition of "acceptable," is different for every woman. In some cases where the patient chooses a lumpectomy, the surgeon is unable to "clear the margins" surgically, that is, remove enough of the tissue surrounding the tumor to ensure no cancer cells are left and still provide an acceptable cosmetic result. If the surgeon is unable to clear the margins after several attempts, a mastectomy is usually needed. Some other reasons to choose a mastectomy can be the presence of tumor in more than one area of the breast, a history of previous radiation to the chest, small breast size, genetic predisposition, or a concern that the cancer may recur locally, among others. The decision needs to be discussed carefully with your surgeon.

With either procedure, the patient will need to have the lymph nodes under the arm evaluated. Most physicians feel that if there are cancerous cells in the lymph nodes under the arm, the cancer may have spread to other parts of the body. Years ago, the only way to tell if the lymph nodes were involved was for the surgeon to remove the majority of the nodes under the arm. Because the lymphatic system helps reabsorb fluid that gets pushed out into the tissues, their removal in some cases led to *lymphedema*, a permanent swelling of the arm. Over time, surgeons came to understand that the entire lymphatic drainage of the arm goes to just a few nodes first before going to the rest, much like a funneling system. With this knowledge, the *sentinel lymph node biopsy procedure* was born. In this procedure, usually two types of dye, a visible blue dye and a radioactive dye, are injected around the tumor or around the nipple. The dye takes the same path a tumor cell might take if it were to break free from the tumor. The dye gets trapped in the first few nodes, or sentinel nodes, that drain the breast. These nodes are then removed and examined for disease. If there is no disease seen in these nodes, there is no need to remove additional nodes under the arm and the risk of lymphedema is greatly reduced.

Continued on page 123

No More Octobers!

Gayle Tanber

I'd been through it all before: the irregular mammogram (also known as "mash-o-gram"), the questions, the biopsy, the results, then nothing to worry about. But this last time was different. Boy was it different! I should have known—it was shortly after the devastation of September 11th. Nothing was the same, nor would it ever be again.

In October I had my annual mash-o-gram, three months late but close enough. They found something that needed to be tested. Been there, done that, so nervous, yes, but not panicked. The amazing thing is I'm not sure they would have ever found it if I hadn't been wearing an uncomfortable bra that day. This particular bra had an underwire that seemed to always bother me on the inside of my left breast, which is why I seldom wore it. But it was nearing laundry day and, well, you know. So, when I was about to be smashed in the vise I asked the tech to pay attention to that one area. Bingo! That's where they found it. Would they have discovered it anyway? Perhaps. At least I would like to think so, but who can say for sure?

It was nearing Christmas before I finally found that it was cancer. My wonderful surgeon tried to tell me that if I were going to get cancer, this was the best kind to get (yeah right!). It was DCIS, an early stage and usually quite curable. Curable my ass, this was *cancer* and I'm scared! What do I do? I'm an intelligent and independent woman, single for so long I've almost forgotten what married life was like (or I blocked it out, not sure which). I figured, I raised two children on my own; if I could handle teenagers I could handle anything.

I wanted to remove the breast but my doctors convinced me it wasn't necessary. There was no lymph node involvement and it was caught pretty early so it was decided just the lump would be removed. I had the surgeon diagram the size and shape of the cancer and include how much surrounding breast would be removed. Then, for whatever reason, I started to get angry about this cancer. I researched my options for hours and hours until I felt I was making informed and reasonable decisions.

No, I decided, I wasn't going to wait until after Christmas to have it removed. (My surgeon still remembers me taking over his appointment book and comparing it to mine so we could agree on a time.) No, I would not use the affiliated oncologist who wouldn't give me direct answers to my questions. His answers of "Just because it's new doesn't mean it's better" and "Because that's been my standard procedure" were totally unacceptable. My feeling of having some control was probably an illusion but it sure made me feel better!

I was determined that this cancer was not going to run my life. I already had a life that I liked, thank you very much. This cancer was going to have to fit into my existing life, which would go on its merry little way. The radiation treatments were just my first appointment of the day and I continued to work, play, hold meetings and conduct my life just as I liked it.

I took the medications recommended, I altered my diet, I continued to work out regularly, I did everything I was supposed to do and life went on—at least for about 10 months. Then here comes October once again and time for another mash-o-gram, a few months late of course. Are you seeing a pattern here? (I personally feel the solution is to simply avoid October from now on.)

You always know when something is up. The technicians try to act cheery and calm as they make excuses why they need to take more films. I've done this too many times. I wish they would just be a bit more honest about it all. I knew right away it wasn't going to be good news, and it wasn't. This time, it was Stage III infiltrating carcinoma in my right breast, the prognosis not nearly so bright. This time the surgeon and all my doctors were moving very fast, quite a reversal from the last time.

The lump was removed, along with more than 24 lymph nodes, but I can't say why it was done that way and why we didn't remove the breast. I don't remember making that decision. I just remember waking up and being surprised it was still there. I was told the upside was no lymph node involvement. The downside: every recurrence is more aggressive than the last and the odds were greater that there will be a next time, will likely involve a major organ and be fatal. I like honesty but that was a bit too honest for me.

I remember thinking for the first time that I was going to die. Alone in front of the computer updating my will, I totally fell apart. I couldn't make myself move or stop crying. I finally made it to my bed and stayed there for nearly 24 hours. I knew my family and friends would be there for me but yet I felt so completely alone. I don't know what woke me from that stupor; I only know something made me decide to fight this cancer one more time. I think anger again played a part as I was recently laid off from my job—coincidence?

So okay, here we go again, same routine, different breast. I figured this had to be the last time; after all, I was out of breasts! If it hit my ass and I needed to remove large portions of that I would be extremely grateful.

I was willing to go through radiation again but I didn't want any part of chemo. I was fighting it all the way but my doctors, friends and family all insisted I should do everything possible, including chemo. I finally gave in and agreed, but I'm still not sure it was the right decision. Lost my toenails, damaged my liver, arthritis in my ankles and knees, the list goes on but what's done is done and the cancer is gone so perhaps it really was the right thing to do.

A friend drove me to my first chemo appointment and another friend picked me up—with a joint in hand. I had no idea so many friends had access to pot. All of a sudden it was being offered by people I would never have suspected would even know how to get it. Of course, my friend the police officer would never understand if he knew that for months he was sitting directly above a small stash. We won't tell.

My birthday party that year was a "Hair Today Gone Tomorrow" party. It just happened to be two weeks after my first treatment and my hair was coming out by the handful. We were at my son's house and made it a family affair. My son shaved my head, my grandson swept up my hair, my daughter styled my wig and my daughter-in-law made me a chocolate birthday cake. As we were sitting at the table eating cake and ice cream, my 4-year-old grandson let me know that was a lot of fun but it was time to put my real hair back on.

Armed with my new wig, I went job hunting, went to networking events, walked in the Fiesta Bowl parade, continued my volunteer efforts, helped a friend plan her wedding and carried on with the holidays and various events as much as I could. One day, as I was preparing for a job interview, I discovered the wig was nowhere to be found. I searched everywhere and remembered the last place I wore it was at my son's house, where I had removed it and put it in my tote bag. Before I had the chance to call, he called me and said, "Mom, I found your hair. You dropped it in the street." I had visions of tread marks running across the top of my head! Thankfully such was not the case.

Finally, I have hair again. Not much of course, very short and curly, but at least it's mine. Or at least I think it is, where did all that gray come from? It wasn't nearly that bad before. And wait! The eyebrows are returning as well but gray there too? Oh lovely, I'm really loving this. Okay, I've dyed my hair before, I'll just do it again. Dark brown is what I used before so it should work again, right? Wrong! What is this ungodly shade of pink on my head? Where the hell did that come from? A couple of hysterical phone calls later, I'm again dying my hair, but this time darkest black. That should work. OH NO! The brightest orange you've ever seen. Bozo would be proud, but I'm certainly not (I was a huge success at my nephew's wedding in my old hometown, attended by friends I hadn't seen since high school). Four weeks later, I finally had a normal hair color again.

This week is the 4-year anniversary of my final chemo treatment and all is well. I no longer feel anxiety and fear whenever I see a doctor. I'm healthy, happy, gainfully employed and once again a little late scheduling my routine mash-o-gram. I figure that's okay though; as long as I avoid October there shouldn't be any problem!

A baby boomer from the Midwest, Gayle Tanber moved to Arizona while married with two children. A few short years later, she found herself a single mother living hundreds of miles away from family but determined to stay in Phoenix. Now the proud mother of two happily married children and grandmother of three, she is still single and loving it, and she is working and playing every chance she gets.

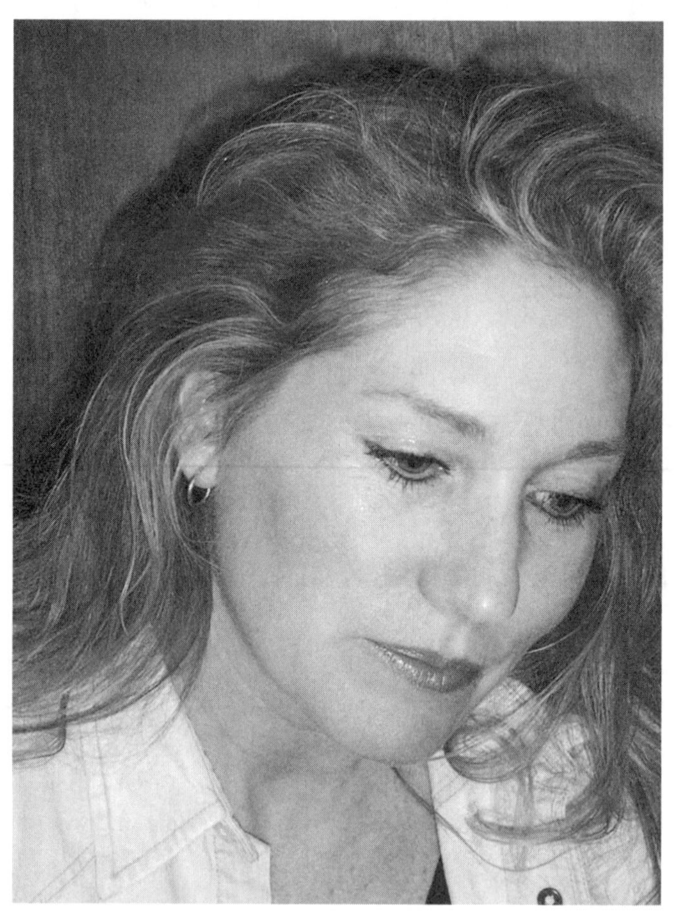

Rene Holly

Pretty Is...Is Pretty Does

(A Praise Poem for Ellie Chandler, Virgie Ruth Everett and Pequita Jo Smith)

Rene Holly

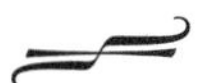

I recall the phrase
my storyteller
of a Grandmother
used to say,
"*Pretty is...is pretty does*,
but ugly goes to the bone."

There was something special
in Maw Maw's logic
which reverberates in my mind and soul....
As I notice the begin of the droop...
as gravity begins to take its toll...
I hear Mama,
"Remember, someone always has it worse than you."

Then I think of Ellie...
the blood drops on her white bra...
the biopsy...the diagnosis—
ductal carcinoma...
the journey from Double D
to nothing...

incisions and stitches running
in half moon lines
resembling closed eyes and lashes
across her chest
where she once had breasts...
the indentations in her flesh
where the drain lines penetrated her sides.
I think of sacrifice...Jesus...
the doubting disciples...
placing their fingertips into His palms.

As she contemplates reconstruction,
I think of resurrection.
As I see her pour the merlot
into a vessel like Christ's chalice,
I flash on working the
blood
down the lines from her sides
into the bulbs...then measuring the output...
cleansing and redressing her wound sites...
until her expanders underneath each
pectoral wall—
gradually, over time—-
    inflate
like hard footballs.
El glares into the mirror,
"Oh, my, I look like Barbie in a train wreck."

I ponder aloud, "What do you mean by that?"

El, with a half smile,
"Didn't you ever peel off Barbie's clothes
and notice they're *not* ana*tom*ically correct—
    no nipples...
and all these scars.
God, I hope they fade."

Subsequently, following another surgery…
when the saline implants take their rightful place…
El says, "Ooh…feel them! Go ahead!
It's okay! They're not real.
        They
        feel
like water balloons."

Later, I think of the Pillsbury Dough Boy
as I view the
        chef
        hats
housing the tender skin
grazed from between her thighs…
which when removed
have formed
her newly coveted nipples
which are perfectly mouth-size.

El admits,
"God, I never knew
how much of my self worth
was tied to my breasts…
but, you know, it's where
        men's eyes
have always gone first.
My friend, do you think anyone
will ever want me again?"
Worry and tears spring to her eyes.

Reassuringly, I answer what I feel to be truth,
"When someone truly loves you,
they will admire *all* that you are…
all that you have lived…
and tenderly kiss your scars.
If they *don't*, they're *not* worth *your* love."

El graciously PRAYS,
"Thank God!
They got all of the cancer...
and I still possess life and breath..."
even though she still *cries* at *times*
for the *loss* of her re*mem*bered *self.*

She now exudes sage-wise mantras:
"I accept my scars as badges of courage...
I have learned to
live from the soul
opposed to in the flesh."
Amazing, the depth that comes from
living
life altering,
body image-dealt deaths.

As for MySelf,
I PRAISE above all else:
Pretty is...IS pretty does...
for I know that my own *beauty*
is not merely *skin deep*
or in vivacious curves' sweep
but it resides in
the *spi*rited
*do*ing
for those in need.

The author is a writer and currently a master's degree candidate in Education at Tennessee State University.

Part IV

HOW DO I DEAL WITH THIS?

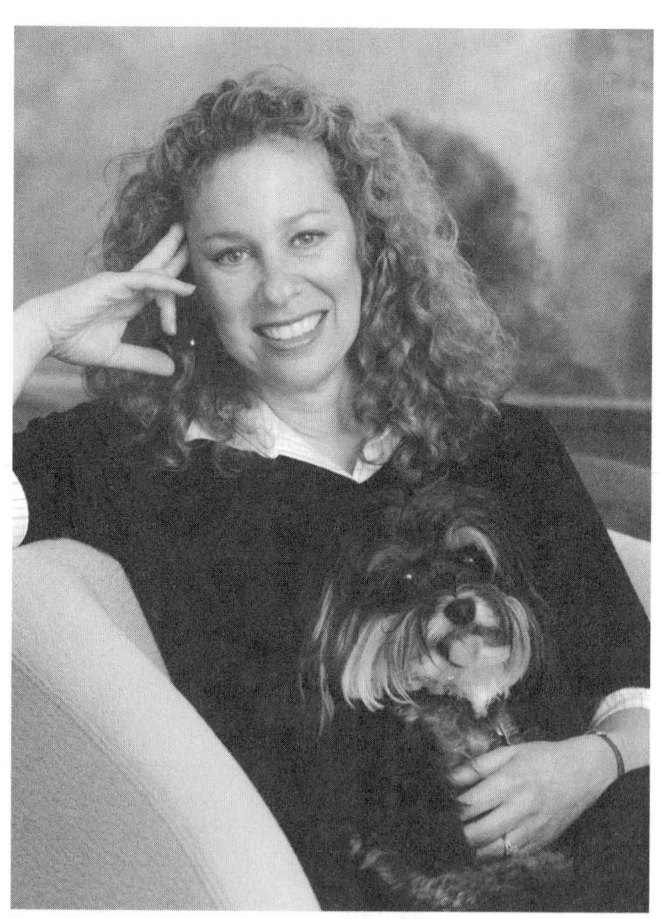

Laney Katz Becker

Breast Cancer and Me: Online and Off

Laney Katz Becker

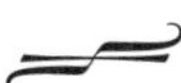

The Place: My house, specifically my bathroom.

The Time: A.M., right after my morning shower.

The Date: Sometime in May, a month before my 39th birthday.

The Event: I was standing naked in front of the mirror, combing through my just-shampooed hair when I noticed a little bump sticking out of the side of my left breast.

Did that catch you by surprise? Because it sure shocked the hell out of me. I still can't believe the lump even caught my eye, it was so tiny. I immediately checked my right breast to see if the itsy-bitsy protrusion was an anatomical thing. It wasn't.

My gynecologist said the lump was nothing to worry about, but sent me to a radiologist, just to be safe. The radiologist saw something called microcalcifications, and send me to a breast surgeon, just to be safe. And the surgeon recommended a biopsy. Just to be safe.

A week after the biopsy (yeah, just to be safe), I returned to the surgeon's office to have my stitches removed. The doctor told me my lump contained some atypical cells but, he said, the lump was completely benign so I needn't be concerned. The only trouble was the surgeon was wrong. Cancer.

Before this official diagnosis, I'd already had a "re" stage: a round of second opinions in which I was *re*evaluated, *re*examined, *re*mammogrammed, and *re*ultrasounded. During this time, I logged onto the Internet looking for information about atypical cells, microcalcifications and breast cancer. That's when I stumbled across the boards. Breast cancer message boards, or bulletin boards, provide opportunities for women to post their thoughts, feelings, questions and yes, even jokes, about every imaginable aspect of the disease. There were women here speaking my language.

My kids were 5½ and 11 years old when I finally received my no-question-about-it diagnosis. I liked the fact that I could read through the boards when the kids were in school and my hubby was at work. And that's what I did at first. I read without contributing. (In cyberspeak that's called lurking.) But after a while I began to post a couple of messages of my own, and later still, I began responding to other women's questions and fears. Once I got involved, I grew to understand what makes this method of communication so great: Location, location, location. It's so convenient; the world is literally at your fingertips.

I loved the fact that I could talk to women who were in my situation without ever leaving my house. I didn't even have to get dressed, which was an added attraction since there were days I was too sick from chemo to even take a shower, let alone don clothes and risk injuring myself or someone else by getting behind the wheel of a car (even without the warning labels on my prescription bottles, I knew better than to even think about operating heavy machinery!).

But convenience of location wasn't the only appeal of the cyberworld. Online boards are available 24/7. The traditional face-to-face support group nearest my home only met once every other week. I was on the message boards *every day*. Also, my local group always met at night, which just happened to be when I was the most tired, the most nauseous, and the most weepy. While I know my decision didn't have to be either/or, the online option just worked so much better for me: it fit my schedule *and* my needs.

At first I felt a little nosy, reading messages, peeking into strangers' lives. But I soon discovered the benefit of sharing: we could all learn from each other's mistakes, prosper from one another's knowledge, and support each other's decisions. This was a place where our feelings could be understood and validated. Some women wrote about their parents' reactions to their cancers, others wanted advice about what to tell their own children. Some women offered prayers, while others offered beauty tips about how best to camouflage the loss of eyebrows and eyelashes. No complaint was too small, we covered it all: foods to eat when mouth sores from chemo made eating nearly impossible, where to find bathing suits for our new, changing and often one-breasted bodies, and what to say to well-meaning friends who asked stupid questions like, "Why do you think you got breast cancer?"

I gathered strength from all the different stories and felt empowered as I read about how other women courageously faced their challenges. In spite of the fact that our ages, lifestyles, sexual orientation, and socio-economic backgrounds represented a true cross-section of America, we had no trouble relating. All of us cyber-strangers had something much bigger in common, and our individual desires for information and support helped unite us as a whole. It was comforting to know we didn't have to go it alone and cyber-ears were always available to listen. Besides, sometimes it was just easier to share and/or face our deepest fears with total strangers.

I was fortunate to have many wonderful friends who helped me through my year of cancer. They cooked meals for me and my family, drove me to and from doctors' appointments, ran errands, and provided rides for my kids. And I had loving family members and a husband who never complained. (I did enough of that for us both.) For me, the boards supplemented what I received in real life.

But not all women are as lucky to have such extensive face-to-face support. That makes the online option that much more important. And, I must admit, as helpful as my friends and family members were, there was something profoundly moving about being able to connect with other women who'd already walked in my shoes. There are some things, I learned, that can only be truly understood by women who have been there, done that. And thanks to the Internet, finding such soulmates is no longer just a possibility, it's a probability.

Laney Katz Becker is an award-winning writer and the author of *Dear Stranger, Dearest Friend*, a novel based on her experience with breast cancer, and *Three Times Chai*, a collection of rabbis' favorite stories. As a journalist, Laney's articles have appeared in more than 50 publications including *Self*, *Seventeen*, *First for Women*, and *Health*. After more than two decades of working as a writer, Laney now works as a literary agent at Folio Literary Management in New York City.

Mints and Mothballs

Caroline Nye

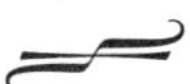

The first ring of the phone roused me from sleep in the darkness of early morning. The second ring caused my insides to curl into a ball with apprehension. By the fourth ring, a tear had already made its way down my cheek. I heard Mum padding down the stairs to answer it. I could tell by the sound of her dragging steps that she didn't want to answer the phone, didn't want to ruin the beautiful stillness of that morning, and our lives, with the news we hoped would never arrive.

Several weeks earlier, we learned my grandmother had been diagnosed with breast cancer. We were invited around to her house as a family and I excitedly entered the welcoming living room, with its familiar smell of mothballs and mints. I didn't notice the preoccupied looks on my grandparents' faces as I headed straight for the bowl of sweets. I was old enough to understand how serious cancer was but also easily reassured that it could be cured; I was also young enough to believe that death could never touch me or anyone else in my family. I looked for signs of illness in my grandmother as she sat quietly in her favorite armchair, something to tell me that this was real and that she was as ill as the sadness in the room suggested. But her face told another story. Her eyes met mine and were calm and comforting. She smiled, told me not to worry, that whatever happened she would be fine. I left with a downcast heart. It must be some kind of a mistake, I thought. She seemed fine.

Her operation went well. I didn't understand all that was done to her but I did understand "recovery." Afterwards, life began to return to normal and I believed that she would soon be well enough to pick me up from school every Tuesday as she always had done. But the following Tuesday I walked home, angry and upset. If she had really recovered, then why wasn't life the same as before?

A week later, my grandparents invited us around again. The bowl of sweets went ignored as I gingerly entered the house and peered at my grandmother, afraid of what I might see. There she sat, in the same armchair, but she didn't look the same. She still smiled warmly and welcomed us in the comforting voice I had known since I was a tiny child. We wrapped our hands around cups of hot chocolate and talked about the things we always used to talk about: school, my parents' work, the cat, my grandfather's roses. But nobody mentioned that her face was thinner, that she lacked the usual color in her cheeks, that there was something distinctly different about her that gave me a sense of sadness I had never experienced before.

It wasn't until we were in the car on the way home that I was told the cancer had spread. The little warm ball of hope I had been holding on to so tightly began to turn cold. I wanted my father to turn the car around and drive back: I realized I hadn't hugged her as tightly as I should have, nor told her how wonderful I thought she was. I was frightened that in all of our years together I had forgotten to tell her how much I appreciated her and everything she had ever done for me and now there might never be time. But we drove on and in voices much less reassuring than before, my parents told me that everything would be alright.

Several days later we were again at my grandmother's house, but my grandmother wasn't sitting with us. Small talk patched the holes in the conversation where silence would have been unbearable. One by one, my parents and older sister climbed the stairs to see my grandmother who, I was told, preferred to stay in bed now. My grandfather gave me sweets and tried to keep me entertained but all I could focus on was the face of each person as they descended the stairs, chewing their lower lips, forcing a smile at one another. Then it was my turn; I had insisted. The advice whispered to me as I slowly walked up the stairs was "try not to cry in front of her, it will make her feel worse." I took a deep breath and then crept in, as if by not making a sound, things would be okay and she would be sitting there, painting or knitting as normal.

My grandmother beckoned me to the bed. "I'm sorry," was all I could say as tears forced themselves out of my eyes and ran down onto her bed. My grandmother was almost unrecognizable as she lay there, even thinner than before, her skin a translucent yellow. But when she smiled, I knew it to be her and I gingerly took her hand. We talked about the usual things for a while, but we both knew this would be the last time we would ever see each other. It was heart-breaking yet beautiful, devastating, but I realized my luck in being able to say goodbye properly and tell my grandmother how much I loved her, and all the things about her which had made me the person I had become and all the things I would remember her for. Her calm serenity put a stop to my tears. I allowed only one more to quietly escape as she weakly squeezed my hand. "I love you," she whispered as I softly closed the door behind me.

So when the phone stopped ringing on that early morning and I heard my mother quietly crying in the kitchen, I knew. We all knew. Yet mixed with the pain, the worry for my grandfather, the sudden, desperate emptiness that shook my body silently on that dark day, was the same sense of calm that my grandmother had managed during that last visit and, in spite of everything, I believed that she, and we, would be alright.

After receiving a degree in social anthropology from Edinburgh University, the author traveled the world while training in organic agriculture, working part time with terminally ill people, and eventually ending up as a wildlife officer in Spain. A published writer, she currently resides in Switzerland.

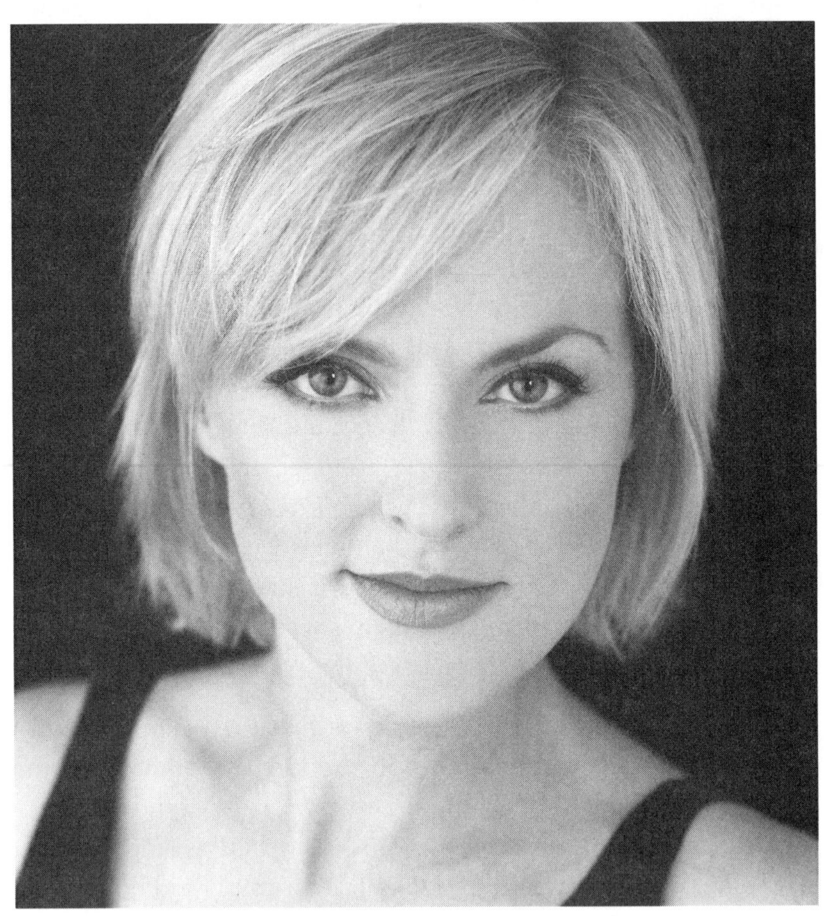

Elaine Hendrix

Thank You Granny Ruth

Elaine Hendrix

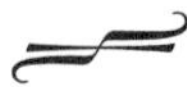

We were sitting on the couch at my father's house enjoying a snack and watching a little television, when out of the complete blue my grandmother asked me, "When are you are going to get married?"

Bug-eyed and nearly choking on my cracker and cheese I asked back, "Married? I don't know. Why?"

"What about your friend Gregg? I like him."

"Well, Gran," I said, pausing briefly and thinking I was stating the obvious, "Gregg is *gay*."

"Oh." Gran sat there and thought about this for a moment. "Well, you could always live together."

Ruth Hodges Hendrix, known to me my whole life as "Granny Ruth" a.k.a. "Gran," was an awesome grandmother—and she was a hoot to say the least. A high school graduate at the age of thirteen, Gran was born and raised in southwestern Kentucky. Always on the go and possessed of a wicked sense of humor, she loved to dance, wrote letters and postcards to me, bought me clothes, and called me on the phone. She took the whole family on yearly trips in her vintage wood-paneled station wagon, entertaining us with an endless supply of stories between playful threats of "chop-popping" and heartfelt refrains of "Rocky Top." She was my most avid supporter and never passed up a chance to brag about me. Who could ask for anyone better to share a part of one's life with? I wouldn't trade it for all the gold in Fort Knox. (Where Gran took us one summer during a family vacation!)

It wasn't until her death in 2004 that I realized she had also been the most constant part of my life. My parents divorced when I was six, and I spent countless hours traveling almost weekly between the households of my divided family—many years between different cities in Tennessee, Kentucky, Georgia, and California. When I grew up I traveled the world, working as a single gal in an extremely unstructured and unpredictable business. Granny Ruth, on the other hand, lived in the same house for 60 years, complete with the same phone number, landscaping and furniture. An elementary school teacher for 25 years, she was married to my grandfather, "Pop Pop Tommy," for over half a century. She was my strongest anchor, my sense of "home."

It had been almost 10 years since Gran was first diagnosed with breast cancer—while caring for her husband, whose undetected prostate cancer had sent an army of other cancers to storm his body. He lay sick for months on end while she cared for him and received her radiation treatments. True to her Great Depression–survivor character, she never complained. Not once.

Now it was Gran's turn. It was January, "pilot season," the beginning of the busiest time of the year for me. I had a recurring role in a hit television show called *Joan of Arcadia* and I was eager for a show of my own. But my dad and his sister had taken as much time as they could to tend to their mother during her rapid downturn over Christmas. I wanted to give them a break and spend some time taking care of my Granny Ruth for what were clearly to be the last days of her life, despite the loose threads of hope and optimism that still dangled around us.

So I, along with my faithful four-legged girl Tiloc, left the fray of Hollywood to spend as much time as needed in little Elizabethtown,

Kentucky. Gran had invited me several times to bring my dog to visit her. I hadn't until that point, though it would have been great fun for Gran. "Why didn't I bring Tiloc sooner?" was skipping in my head like a scratched record. The question might have plagued me for the rest of my life had it not been for my father and the rest of my family, who reminded me that we were there now, and that's what mattered. Gran taught them well. She would have said the very same thing.

When I first arrived at Gran's that January, she could walk to the bathroom with some assistance. By the end of the week she could not leave her bed. We had the amazing assistance of hospice care workers and in-home caretakers, but I insisted on taking care of as much as I possibly could. I sat with Gran the entire time, playing big band music, watching TV with her, feeding her baby food, monitoring her every shift and groan and, most importantly, hugging her when the morphine's hallucinations got too "real" for her. The two weeks I spent with her were extraordinary. It was a great honor, a privilege and a gift to be able to tend to the woman who had loved me, her only granddaughter, so deeply.

Gran's battle with cancer (ultimately ovarian) ended in the very same room in which Pop Pop Tommy's fight with cancer had ended nine years before—almost to the day. The last of the family had left just that morning, as if Gran had waited to let everyone near and dear to her say a final farewell. Later in the evening, with no one there but the night nurse and myself, I stood beside my Granny Ruth and watched her take her last breath on this earth. My gratitude for the opportunity to be with her at the end surpassed all that is sacred in this world.

My Aunt Alice was also diagnosed with breast cancer, but she luckily got it in time. My dad caught his prostate cancer early and nipped it in the bud. My grandfather on my mother's side died of an extremely rare heart cancer. I have other family members who have made their crossing via the big "C," so I am well aware that

I will need to stay on top of it myself, since it runs so rampant in my genes on both sides.

That's OK though. We all have a number, and when it's called, that's it. My days with Granny Ruth taught me that life is short and very precious, but not so short that you can't appreciate even the "last minutes," and not so precious that you can't have a lot of good hearty laughs along the way. My gratitude for having had this experience with her is boundless. I think about it regularly and am constantly reminded of what is truly important about it all: love and connection. Thank you, Granny Ruth. You gave me so much both during and after your life. I love you and I miss you tremendously.

Oh, and as of this writing, I'm still not married...and Gregg is still gay. Say "hi" to Pop Pop for me.

Elaine Hendrix (*The Parent Trap*, *What the Bleep Do We Know?!*, *Joan of Arcadia*) is an award-winning film and television actress, established singer/songwriter, classically trained dancer, veteran film and stage producer, published author, avid animal activist, and *rabid* Tennessee Volunteer. Is there a term for someone who takes "triple-threat" to a whole new level? What about...*Superstar!*

Elaine has particular affinities for vanilla ice cream, *Star Wars*, Elvis and Target and believes it is important to maintain a healthy balance of work, play, spirituality and shopping in her life. She lives in Los Angeles with her entertainment attorney boyfriend Christopher J. Corabi and their four rescued animals: canines Tiloc and Rossmore, and felines Goodie Cornbread and Kimbo.

Officially find her at www.elainehendrix.com and www.myspace.com/elainehendrix.

Connecting

Peggy Duffy

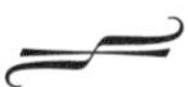

One night, three months after moving with my husband and three children from New Jersey to Virginia, I answered the phone and was greeted by Roseanne's familiar New York accent. Our calls before Christmas were a long-standing tradition and, in my still-unfamiliar environment, I looked forward to sharing the comfort and intimacy that comes with years of friendship. Roseanne was the last connection to my youth, the only friend I'd kept in touch with from high school. Physical distance could never unravel the closeness that years of intimate confessions had knit together.

"I have so much to tell you," she began.

While I settled into easy-listening mode, expecting an update on her job or her three children, she announced she was recovering from brain surgery. I heard "brain tumor" and "cancer." For the next two hours, she poured it out—her physical symptoms, the operation, the radiation and steroid treatments she was in the middle of, the chemotherapy that would soon follow. Her doctors determined that the cancer had originated in her breast and spread to her brain, but due to the type of cancer, they hadn't done a mastectomy. I didn't know what to say, which made her laugh. "I've never known you to be speechless before," she said.

Although it was well past midnight, when I hung up with Roseanne I promptly called my friend Barb in New Jersey. I needed someone to talk to and she is an oncology nurse.

"It's in her brain?" she asked in a voice I didn't like.

"Yes. What's her prognosis?" I asked. I *had* to know.

"I'm only telling you this because you asked," she said. "She's not going to make it. For reasons we don't understand yet, when cancer metastasizes from the breast to other parts of the body, we can't stop it. If she lives," she added, "she'll earn a spot in the *Guinness Book of World Records*."

Barb went on to explain in her best nurse's voice how each time chemotherapy is administered, it cuts the number of cancerous cells in half. But no matter how many treatments a patient receives, the laws of mathematics tell us there will always be a few remaining cells. In many cancers, those cells remain dormant and the patient stays in remission. She told me Roseanne could go into remission for awhile, but the cancer would come back, and it would grow faster and more vigorously.

Barb did not give me the details of the treatment, treatment that in the beginning—before the disease really grips with its ravaging claws—is worse than the disease. But Roseanne did. In the months that followed, she chronicled both the debilitating progression of a frightfully invasive disease and her battle against it. Her brain was radiated. She took steroids which kept her awake most of the night. She was injected with lethal chemicals she could taste in her mouth and smell in her sweat. She wanted strawberries or melons, anything juicy and sweet, but the chemo weakened her immune system and raw fruit had too much bacteria. She grew weak. She lost weight. She lost her hair.

We never discussed her prognosis. She wouldn't have believed her doctors even if she'd asked them. She preferred her own prognosis: she would get well. She was full of hope, inspired and supported by family and friends both near and far. And she had her religion: a revitalized faith in God and the Catholic Church made stronger with each more desperate day.

That summer, things began to look up. She was officially in remission. Round one of chemotherapy was over. Her doctors advised her to forget about the cancer for a while. Take a vacation. Enjoy her family. She did.

In the fall, she resumed chemotherapy and was still considered cancer free. There was talk of a bone marrow transplant. It would mean a hospital stay over the Christmas season in a semi-isolated, sterile room.

Roseanne would talk to me and I would talk to Barb. I passed along this newest development about the bone marrow transplant. "Will it work?" I asked, hoping this might keep her cancer free. "It won't make her well. Or cure her. One never gets over cancer, like a cold or the flu, one just prays to remain cancer free. It might work, but it's risky. There's a good chance she would die on the table."

Did Roseanne know that, I wondered. She was so reluctant to leave her children, so torn between undergoing the transplant and being home that year for Christmas. After the insurance company refused to pay for the procedure because, at the time, it was still considered experimental, she talked more and more of the risks involved. She felt her doctors were only interested in her as a statistic, another number in the success or failure column. Was it fear or relief that made her react with such anger?

I was swept up in her anger, I echoed it, fed it. Together, we directed it at her doctors, but I realize now that she had turned her anger inward and now blamed herself for the disease, because the cancer came back with a vengeance. It had never really gone away. Her new oncologist, a kind and gentle man who launched her on a new round of chemotherapy, tried to reassure her that she had done nothing to bring on this disease. He explained the unusually aggressive nature of her cancer, which continued to defy treatment despite the high toxicity of the chemicals they used.

That second year, her life approached normalcy. Our phone discussions included our kids, mutual friends and her job (which she now did from home). The cancer became a part of her existence. She'd be hospitalized a few days each month, sedated, and administered her chemotherapy. Then she'd return home and resume her life. This stage didn't last long.

The disease invaded new tissue and grew. The doctors removed one of her breasts. She told me she had open sores on the other that incessantly oozed and tumors which covered her back. When I called the third Christmas after her diagnosis, her mom answered the phone. "She's in the hospital, but she'd love to hear from you," she said. Roseanne and I didn't talk long. Struggling to breathe, she said the cancer was in her lungs.

It was after the New Year when I heard from her again and she was openly scared. She'd found out no one had expected her to leave the hospital. "They put me in here to die," she said, an audible quiver in her voice. All optimism was gone. She'd given up on the idea of beating the disease or ever resuming a normal healthy life. But she could live with the debilitation, the weakness and the disfigurement, as long as she would live. She was willing to accept this cycle of hospitalization and treatment and sickness forever.

"I have three very good reasons to live," she said, and we cried together at the thought of her three children. She tried to make me laugh over what little was left to laugh about. Like how she had no hair left anywhere on her body, except for her legs. "You'd think I could have been spared still having to shave them," she said to fill the silence between our tears.

As soon as I hung up the phone that day, I called Barb. "How do you do what you do," I asked bitterly, "surrounded by death every day?"

"It isn't easy," she admitted. "All I can do is help my patients accept their own death. Not all of them can."

I never helped Roseanne face her death. I avoided the truth, encouraging her with my silence, grateful for the phone because she couldn't see my face. I never even went to see her. It seems unfathomable to me now; she was only five hours away by car. But she never asked, and though I said a number of times, "If you need anything…" I never insisted. It was as if we both sensed my seeing her would confirm the reality neither of us wanted to face.

Roseanne had once been a very private person, confiding her personal thoughts and feelings to only an intimate few. Toward the end, she became open and emotional, raw and exposed.

"They are using the word terminal now," she informed me in one of our last conversations. "I do not like that word."

She called me another night around nine o'clock. It was not a time we usually spoke anymore. I heard her husband and kids in the background. She was laughing one minute and crying the next. There was no single thread that ran through her words, but rather a messy tangle of thoughts. That sense of looking toward the future with either hope or acceptance was gone, replaced by this helpless hysteria.

"Morphine," she explained amid her ramblings, though she didn't know she was explaining anything. "They have me on morphine now. I'm stoned out of my mind."

It was the very last time I heard her voice. I wish I'd known that at the time. A week later, she died. She'd been sick for close to three years. She was thirty-eight years old.

I can't help but think about the pain there must have been toward the end. Pain she never once complained about. How would I have coped?

Naturally with her line of work, Barb had asked herself the same question. "I wouldn't do it," she had said to me during one of our calls. "If I had cancer, I'd live the best I could as long as I could. I wouldn't treat it."

"How can you say that?" I asked, surprised. "It's prolonged Roseanne's life."

"But look at her quality of life," She replied. "I wouldn't want to live like that."

At the time, I believed her. I think she believed it herself. It sounds hard, but she didn't say it that way.

Not long after Roseanne died, Barb called and told me she'd found a lump in her breast. "I didn't want to tell you before, because I didn't want you to worry," she said. "But I had it removed and everything's fine. It was benign."

She gave me the details of the discovery, the biopsy and the long wait for the results. "The wait was awful," she said. "Because of my work, I knew too much. I knew all the possible treatments and what my chances would be. Sometimes, ignorance is bliss."

As I listened, it wasn't a nurse's voice I heard. Behind the sound of confidence and competence was that same desperate, clinging-to-life-at-all-costs sound that I had heard in Roseanne's.

"I know I said that I wouldn't treat it, but I don't feel that way any more," she confessed. "I would do whatever I had to."

I heard those words with a sense of relief, a reaffirmation that what holds us here is so strong that no one can easily let go of it.

Peggy Duffy's short stories and essays have appeared in numerous publications, including *Newsweek*, *The Washington Post*, *The Christian Science Monitor*, and *Notre Dame Magazine*, as well as various anthologies including *Cup of Comfort for Mothers to Be* and *Cup of Comfort for Mothers and Sons*. One of her short stories was selected by *storySouth* for the Million Writers Award, Notable Online Short Stories for 2004, and two of her stories were selected by *storySouth* as Notable Online Short Stories for 2003.

Continued from page 92

Chemotherapy

Chemotherapy for breast cancer usually involves a combination of drugs that kill tumor cells in the breast and, more importantly, cells that may have traveled elsewhere. Chemotherapy is *cytotoxic*, meaning that the drugs will work to kill any rapidly dividing cells in the body, whether or not they are cancerous. This explains many of the side effects experienced by patients such as hair loss, decreased red and white blood cell count and gastrointestinal symptoms (cells that line the intestines grow relatively rapidly). The drugs may be given intravenously, by mouth or by injection, and usually in cycles, in order to allow the body to recover from their effects. There are many combinations and classifications of drugs available and the best course of treatment needs to be chosen in consultation with your *medical oncologist*, the doctor responsible for helping you make decisions regarding chemotherapy.

Endocrine therapy can be used by patients with cancers that have receptors for estrogen and progesterone. Therapies can include tamoxifen, *aromatase inhibitors* in post-menopausal women, or *ovarian ablation*, drug therapy to suppress the production of estrogen. Herceptin® is a drug that works as an *antibody*. The drug attaches to the receptor created by the HER2 gene and marks the cell for destruction. There are newer drugs being developed that will target cancers that over-express the HER2 gene, offering more hope to women with this aggressive form of disease. Again, the specific agent and length of treatment need to be discussed with your medical oncologist.

What is very important to remember when considering potential therapies is that each patient is an individual and what works with one patient may not work with the next. Also, remember that there are choices involved in treatment planning and there may be more than one path a patient can choose regarding her therapy. You need to discuss your choices carefully with your doctors and, if needed, seek more than one opinion about the treatment to be used.

Continued on page 146

It Doesn't Have To Be About Fighting

Judy Gordon

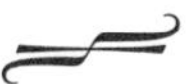

I chose an uncommon way to cope with the diagnosis and treatment of breast cancer. I wasn't a warrior, as many cancer patients and survivors describe themselves. I didn't see cancer as something to wage a battle against. But surrender might be too strong a word to describe what I did. "Going with the flow" is more accurate.

To begin with, I fell apart. The conventional "stay positive" wisdom didn't work for me. I couldn't fight my way through. I wasn't any good as a fighter. My oncologist told me that patients who fall apart are more likely to rebuild their lives better once they are through the rough treatments. Did she say that just to give me validation and encouragement, or was it truly her experience? As I reflected in my journal, *"If you don't experience your emotional response in the moment, you will experience it at some future time."*

Falling apart was what I needed to do for myself, but it was hard on others, at least in the beginning. I couldn't be Judy-as-usual. As I went through the process of giving in to my fears, I became unpredictable. Suddenly, I was no longer positive nor upbeat nor optimistic. I had no "go-for-it spirit" even though I was constantly reading and hearing that a go-for-it spirit was a requirement. I was showing a different side that was a creation of the experience, and I needed to be authentic to that creation.

My reactions to treatment took many turns. While I despised feeling physically ill, the emotional turmoil hit me harder and I told people how it was going with me, whatever it was that was going on, and that seemed to demystify the cancer experience for them. Even in this day and age, when we all know people who have or have had cancer, the emotional experience of the illness is not well understood. Although I might have scared some people with my tell-all attitude, some told me they appreciated my candor: they always knew how I was feeling and what I needed, and that made them feel more involved.

It also allowed some friends to open up about cancer experiences in their own lives. People who had experienced cancer themselves told me things that helped me the most. They were my role models, and I learned a lot from them. Someone three months ahead of me in treatment advised me to "just do it one day at a time." A childhood friend who had experienced breast cancer and subsequent prophylactic mastectomies counseled me: "You just keep feeling better after awhile and then you forget how bad you felt." Another told me, "You can get through it, and you will." They spoke of what they knew to be true; their statements were not necessarily profound or revelatory, but they were real and they resonated with me.

Even though I fell apart, I didn't completely lose my sense of fun. A bright side of treatment was, literally, a red wig. Even before my short, wavy, black-hair-streaked-with-gray fell out, I bought a wig that looked very similar to my own hair. But once it was gone, I actually preferred wearing scarves for public appearances and a small cotton cap for around the house. Near the end of my chemo treatment, though, I made a bold change. Gazing at the wigs in my oncologist's office, wigs that previous patients had donated for others' use, my husband and I were attracted to a red one. I didn't need any encouragement to try it on. Even without a stylist's adjustment, it looked good. We took it! The first time friends saw me wearing it, they were startled. People commented on how much they liked it, and I took that to heart. It was fun to be different, to surprise people (and myself), and to look better. It also gave me the opportunity to be lighter and freer. Six months later, when my own hair was growing back, it was actually difficult to give up wearing the wig.

As recovery progressed, a powerful, positive sensation hit me. I had survived an awful experience. My worst fears were not realized and the experience hadn't lasted forever. It was not quite a feeling of being "Superperson," but it was super-amazing to me that normalcy returned. It is wonderful to learn what we can cope with, even if we fall apart during the journey.

In the beginning, when my husband and I were in a crash learning course on the disease, I read a lot about other people's cancer journeys and professional advice for people on cancer journeys. Most would say that cancer is life-changing in a positive way, and that you have to "give up something in order to receive." Before you've actually gone through such an experience, these words are not very helpful; they sound terribly trite and self-servingly noble. And yet, once you are through this difficult, you can't help but value, celebrate, and learn something from them. Whether we let ourselves recognize the gifts we get from hardship is a matter of attitude.

I am glad I chose my own path to follow on my cancer journey. I know that previous generations were more likely to keep personal challenges to themselves. But I have let my breast cancer experience flow out of me through my writing, in conversations, in correspondence, and in visible emotions and I feel healed in many ways. My future is not guaranteed, but I see it differently now. And I believe my story is an example of openness and authenticity that others may find helpful.

A young friend wrote this to me during the course of my treatments: "Sometimes we need to see other people do something that's scary first and then we can start to step into the unknown ourselves. So many times we are asked to 'let go' in order to grow, but we can't because we're afraid. Your experience into the unknown and of surrendering to forces out of your control is a miracle and something to be shared." I write this for those who may some day be on such an unwelcome journey themselves.

Judy Gordon is a freelance writer of how-to publications for nonprofit clients. She has more than 25 years' experience in nonprofit management and program development. This story is an excerpt from the book she and her husband co-authored, *The Heroics of Falling Apart: One Couple's Breast Cancer Journey*. She and her family live in Denver, Colorado.

The Glamorous Grandmother

Erica Rivera

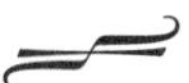

My grandmother, even at seventy, was never an old lady. She lived on the top floor of a senior high-rise in Bloomington, just a little closer to heaven than the rest of the residents. She was never one of them, the fuddy-duddies who congregated in the common room, playing Parcheesi on plaid-covered couches by the fireplace. My grandmother was gorgeous—a wrinkled, bronzed, brunette version of Marilyn Monroe. Her hair, always salon perfect; her nails, always lacquered scarlet; her scent, always Elizabeth Arden Red Door; her breath, always spearmint. She wore pearls—big, brushed, white baubles—like a halo that had slipped over her head and landed around her neck, come to rest on the fuzzy collars of her sweaters.

When the weather was warm we'd trek to Southtown Mall. Despite lifelong diabetes, she was unwilling to starve her sweet tooth and we'd load up on sugar-free caramels at Fannie Mae. My grandmother was also the quintessential bargain hunter; shopping the sale racks was a sport for her.

On special occasions we'd lunch with the geriatric crowd at Red Lobster. While waiting for a table, I'd stare at the lobsters bobbing in the tanks, my childhood brain unable to accept that those little beings would soon be on someone's plate.

"Why are these ones brown?" I asked one day.

"Uh…they're just a different kind of lobster," Grandma said.

Sometimes we'd go to the musty old General Cinema to take in a movie. And sometimes my favorite place: the grassy knoll behind the high rise, where we'd go "just to roll."

But one day the games stopped and, overnight, I grew up.

I sit down in a hard green chair next to my mother in the sterile treatment room.

My beige sweater is too big. In an attempt to erase the Goodwill stink off it, I washed it, then hung it up to dry. I did not know that sweaters should never be hung, especially not when damp. Now, sticking my fingers in the stretched armholes, I think of all the things I have left to learn. Things of adulthood, like ironing, like washing delicates. Like dying.

My grandmother is perched on the table across from me, sheathed in a starched hospital gown. The doctor enters: a blur of dark hair, a whoosh of white coat featuring an impressive ink stain in the front pocket. I am only eleven, but I immediately regard him as too young to be treating something as ominous as cancer.

He does not waste time on small talk. Instead, he launches into surgical speak and scribbles on a whiteboard on the wall. Words in black marker, organs in red. The drawings are no more comprehensible than his prognosis. His voice is muffled and hollow, as though it were passing through an empty can from a far distance, his terminology a string of unintelligible nonsense. All three of us nod, too polite to ask questions, not wanting to interrupt the suave M.D.

In the time it takes for the doctor to explain how my grandmother's body is infested with tumors, how what was once confined to the breast has moved on to the liver, I have pulled my sleeves so loose that they dangle like paralytic limbs from my body. I roll them up, tucking my arms behind me so my mother does not notice what I've done.

The doctor rattles off a few more terms, a death sentence of around six months perhaps, and is gone as swiftly as he entered. The door takes its time to near the jamb, then clicks shut. Silence blooms between us like an ugly cloud. My mother rubs my grandmother's back in wide circles, their heads bowed together.

"Erica," my mother whispers. I look up, frightened by the similarity in their faces, a resemblance I hadn't noticed before. "How are you doing with all of this?" My expression slackens to mirror theirs, though I don't know what I am supposed to feel.

I don't want to upset them, but I can see in their expectant eyes that they want a reaction. I guess I should act upset, even if I don't understand what is happening. I force a few tears through the corners of my eyes, the inauthentic wetness rolling down my cheeks, which are blazing scarlet with embarrassment.

"I'll be okay," I mutter. My grandmother opens her arms to me and I fold into them, inhaling the Red Door perfume, my head between squishy breasts. Breasts that are killing her.

She got so sick so quickly. She was sent away to the nursing home where nuns with heavy black habits floated to and from her bedside like angels of death. I remember visiting her once and not recognizing my glamorous grandmother buried beneath an avalanche of blankets. Her face was pale and unpainted, her hair thin and flat. I don't remember her words; I remember the stroke of her rough, twiggy fingers across my forehead, a smile that seemed to require enormous effort. Walking back to the car on one of the last sunny afternoons of summer, I knew I would not see her again.

My grandmother passed on an early September morning, specific in her last wishes: that her ashes be scattered on the beaches of Florida. I visited those beaches with my six-month-old daughter and then-husband years later; when we returned home, I discovered I was pregnant with another baby girl. I couldn't help but think that Grandma had something to do with it. She would have adored great-granddaughters.

I honor my grandmother in small ways now: I breast-fed my babies, I run Race for the Cure with her name pinned to my back, I do monthly self-exams, I exercise and eat well in the hopes that I can curb my chances of getting breast cancer. Most importantly, I write about her in the hopes that awareness will inspire everyone to work toward a cure and enable more women to live long lives, cancer free.

The author received a Bachelor of Arts degree from Macalester College and has worked as a counselor in the social services sector, both in domestic violence shelters and treatment centers for children and teens. She was the first place winner of the Poetry Prize at the Powderhorn Writer's Festival in 1997.

Grief Walking

Pauline D. Michel

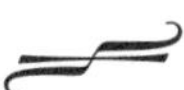

"I have to go for a walk!" The words fly out of my mouth during dinner.

"Where are you going?" asks my youngest son as I get up from the table. I have no answer. I just need to feel the path under my feet, taking me to another place.

There are walks that take you away from something. That is the kind of walking I am doing these days, since my best friend Grier was diagnosed with breast cancer. She is not ready to die and I am not ready to let her go and so we fight together. We fight by staying close, by touching more than ever, looking at each other full in the face and weeping at how our lives have changed without our permission.

So tonight, rather than weep, I go for a walk. I figure that if I move, get some air and enough space, maybe I won't choke to death on this rock in my throat—a rock of anger, pain, disbelief, mistrust, fear and sorrow. I am empty and yet so full of love for her that I am silenced. It hurts to speak her name, but I can speak no other.

"Why is she walking?" asks my middle son as I go upstairs to change into my walking clothes.

"Where is Mom walking *to*?" whispers the youngest.

"She needs to move," answers the oldest.

Since Grier's diagnosis I have been walking every day and often more than once. I feel the pull of the walk coming on. It is like a wave that starts in my stomach and builds in fits and starts until I feel as though I am stuffed with something that wants desperately to get out.

Upstairs I change clothes, wash my face, brush my teeth. I see our picture on my bureau as I pass by from the bathroom. We are outside under the trees in her backyard; tall firs, strong and dark and grown. She is in a playpen. We are both in cloth diapers, barefooted, bare-chested, fair-skinned. Grier with blond hair, fair and silky, sparse and still that of a baby. I am redheaded with hair already thick and full and curly at the ends. I am so much larger than she is. With tiny hands holding on, her mouth just reaches the rail; she bites it. I am standing on my own, my right hand balanced just above her left, poised to touch her with my finger. Only inches separate our noses. Face to face even then, we are mesmerized, caught, joined for life. This is how we have always been: together and open and bare to one another. I keep this photo where I can see it, always.

Outside as I begin my walk, my internal conversation is mainly about what is falling apart in my life. Why do I feel like I have been deserted? This thought catapults me into high speed. The cloudless sky, miles of emptiness above me, matches the emptiness I feel inside. My arms and legs begin to work together; my breathing becomes even and smooth. This is the zone, the walker's high, endorphins on the loose. I must have this every day; I think about it before work, during work, I cannot wait to get to it. Walking has become my tonic.

As the path speeds by under my feet, I am talking out loud to myself, a conversation with Grier about our life together. I see us in a quick succession of snapshots; digging to China in the sand pile in her side yard; climbing up her kitchen counter to reach the candy cupboard; jumping off the side porch as our mothers drink iced tea with orange juice. I see clearly the sleepovers at her house. I see us designing floor plans for our future house out of raked leaves. I see us planning an excursion to the schoolyard, where we had our choice of swings, seesaws, and jungle gyms. A decade later, we would climb to the roof of that school with boys.

After three lumpectomies, Grier decides to part with her breast in the summer and be back at the pool with the kids in time to catch most of their swim meets. I attend the pre-op appointment with her in Philadelphia. Our ride there is like any other. We talk of the kids and husbands. We miss the exit, laughing over her son's recent remark about her approaching mastectomy. She had gathered her four children together to explain what she and her doctors had decided.

"They are going to take off my breast and give me another," Grier told them.

"Will it be a new one or a used one?" Max asked.

"I hope it will be a new one, Max," she answered, trying not to laugh.

We park as close as possible to Pennsylvania Hospital, gather her referral papers, legal pad for note taking and our water bottles. As we cross the street hand in hand I say softly, "Come on Grier, let's go get you a *new* breast."

Inside the hospital, we meet the surgeon.

"Hi Dr. New Breast," Grier says. "This is my friend Paula. She goes with me everywhere and protects me. So be careful."

He looks at me with some apprehension and begins to explain the procedure. He asks Grier to lift her shirt. With a kiss blown to me, she bares her still beautiful, tanned, perfect, size B cups. He weighs them together in his hands and we grin, lifting our eyebrows. He asks to see her stomach, which is flat, tight, and tanned the exact color of her breasts. He gathers what little belly fat there is and pulls a little. We start to laugh and he pauses and smiles cautiously.

"I think you have enough fat here to move up and make another breast," he states.

"Oh, thank you, doctor," Grier says.

He explains that after surgery her belly will be even flatter.

"Do you mean concave?" I ask with disgust.

Grier's surgery goes well. But as the cooler nights arrive and summer wanes, so does she. She spends most of her time on the couch. I notice her voice getting smaller, fainter. Meals are delivered to her home on a regular schedule by neighbors and family. The constant presence of people in her home is a comfort to her and a nuisance to me. I have to sit, watchful and quiet, waiting my turn to join her on the couch to rub her legs and feet. Hypervigilant, I stay close and watch for signs that she has had enough. Grier will look my way and I have permission to clear the house of visitors. I stand guard at her bed and front door. I screen the endless calls. We take long naps together in the quiet of the empty house. My heart breaks over and over as I listen to Grier talk quietly to her four young children about the everyday events of a family.

Since I'm always the one to call her, my heart stops when Grier calls me on a Saturday morning.

"What does asthma feel like?" she asks in a voice I have never heard.

"Why?"

"I can't breathe."

"Grier, how long has this been going on and what did the doc say?"

"I haven't talked to him," she whispers through the start of tears. "I don't want to know."

"You have to call him. You have to find out what this is. Call now," I order.

"What if it's the cancer? And I have these little bumps all over my chest! Maybe it's from the radiation. Do you think?"

"Call him now!"

Monday afternoon, as I drive home from work, she calls with the news I already know in my heart.

"It's in my lungs."

"What is the next step and when do you go?"

"This is different. He said it's a very aggressive kind. There is nothing they can do now."

Then the silence sits with us.

"I don't want to leave you, Paula."

"You never will. I'm on my way."

She is with her husband when I arrive. I have never seen this look of fear, of terror, on her face. It strikes me down. Neither of us speaks as we hold each other and cry.

Fall makes way for winter and Christmas, Grier's favorite season. Her cousins and children put up the tree and decorations. Hers is always a busy home at Christmas, but this year the visitors double in number as word spreads and they come to say goodbye. Holding myself still and silent is the only way to keep myself from shattering. I am losing my friend of fifty years, my mother, my child, my sister, my other self.

I have been with her through the afternoon, through the visitors, hospice workers, her children moving in and out of the living room where she sleeps to be around all those she loves. Kissing the top of her head to say goodnight, I feel what is left of my heart break.

Tomorrow I will walk again. I will find a new road to travel, taking Grier along wherever my fresh path leads. She will walk with me as she always has and we will be together still.

Pauline Michel is a social worker in child welfare for the State of Pennsylvania. She has a master's degree in counseling and has worked in the fields of reproductive technology, adoption and elementary education.

An Autumn Gift

Linda O'Connell

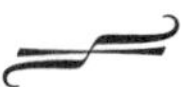

At 51, my friend Rose sported a cockeyed wig and a raspy voice, the result of the debilitating cancer which had robbed her of her hair and her strength. She had more bad days than good, and as the weather cooled, the dark, wet skies mirrored her situation. But after nearly a week, the clouds lifted and so did Rose's spirits. When I came for a visit, she was alert, her voice halting but strong and assertive for a change.

"Take me outside. I want to sit in the sunshine."

She shuffled into the yard with her oxygen tank in tow. We sat in silence, side by side under the sugar maple tree, enjoying the brisk breeze. I tucked her afghan around her. Hundreds of orange, gold and yellow leaves rained down on us and made Rose smile. Memories of our twenty-five-year friendship whirled in our minds like the leaves overhead. We were entranced by the waltzing leaves as wind gusts swept them up and sent them dancing at our feet. The yard was very much alive and so was Rose that day.

"Will you please get me that red leaf," she asked, "and that yellow one?" She pointed here and there, and I bounded about gathering brilliant orange, red and golden yellow leaves into a huge bouquet. Rose tired and asked to go inside. I placed her leaf bouquet on a table beside her, tucked her in and told her I'd see her the next afternoon.

When I arrived the next day, she was glassy-eyed and weak. "I have something for you," she said, pausing breathlessly between words. "Do you remember the big maple tree in the old neighborhood?"

When we were neighbors, the gorgeous towering tree, Mother Nature's masterpiece, was the focal point of our neighborhood each autumn. We were blessed to have it right outside our doors. We collected leaves with our children when they were young and we made centerpieces with the colorful array that carpeted our lawns and sidewalks.

"I made you a gift." She handed me ten sheets of white paper on which she had arranged the colorful leaves that she had selected the day before.

Tears welled in our eyes. "Do you like them? Can you use them?" she asked.

"Yes, I love them and I will treasure them forever," I said.

Like the autumn leaves, Rose completed her life cycle at the end of fall. I laminated the colorful leaf collages, and every year I use them as a teaching aid with my preschool students. And I think of Rose as I tell my students about them.

"Leaves are like people, they come in all shapes, sizes and colors. Trees have roots. Redwood trees are the tallest, and their roots intertwine. They support each other when the strong winds blow, sort of like when you hold hands with your best friend and it makes you feel safe."

This simple treasure is a priceless gift bequeathed with love and it will keep on touching lives, just as my friend Rose did.

An early childhood educator for 30 years, Linda O'Connell is now a freelance writer and writing teacher whose work has appeared in many anthologies, magazines, literary reviews and newspapers. She is inspired by autumn leaves and water; the ocean tugs at her Midwest soul.

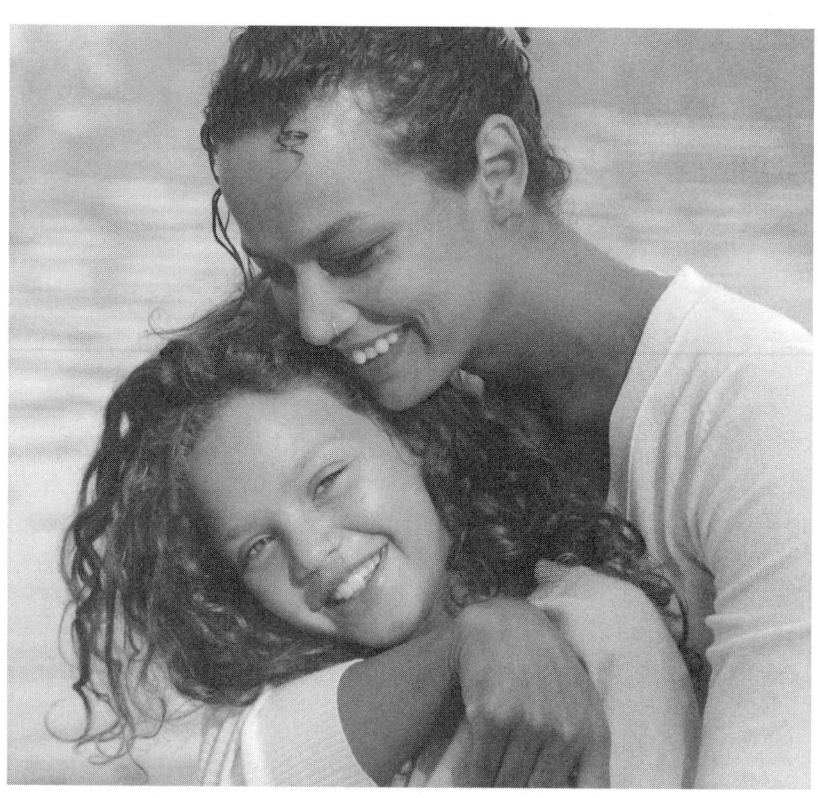

Lorena Perera-Smith

Summer in Sweden

Lorena Perera-Smith

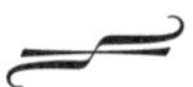

I don't like the smell of cigarettes that much in the U.S., but strangely in Europe it makes me think of summer. I think it's because that smell is on the air when the café terraces open for the summers. People who have been shut in for the winter spill out onto the sidewalks and lounge outside the cafés, drinking coffee and beer and smoking cigarettes in the sun. They push their chairs back, tilt their faces to the sun and let its rays soak into their bones. Over there, cigarettes are the smell of summer.

Today I walked around streets that I hadn't seen for ten years. I took my coffee out to one of the terraces and sat there watching the people walk by, buy flowers in the town square, cycle in the sunshine. The coffee in this particular shop is so good. Or maybe it's the atmosphere that makes it so. I sit here drinking my hot coffee, counting seconds, minutes, hours.

I have come back to this country because my mother is sick. She has cancer. I am sitting here because she is at the hospital getting chemicals pumped into her system, chemicals that are supposed to make her better. The treatments make her lose her hair and move like an old woman.

I stare unseeingly into my magazine and wonder how this could have happened. The model on the page in front of me stares back with pouty lips and flawless skin and I want to dig my nails into her perfect face and rip the page to shreds. I see a young girl coming out of the café holding a drink. She glances at me and I wonder what she sees. A tired woman, circles under her eyes, in dirty jeans and a spotty T-shirt?

Ten years isn't that long but I feel old. Old and tired. I don't think there is anything left of that girl in me. She was beautiful and optimistic and happy. I think, I'm too young to feel this damn old! And smile, because I sound like a song. I think that is a song isn't it? A country song.

Every time I hold my mother's head as she throws up after chemo I feel that girl slip away a little more. When I see her strength fade and her hands tremble, I feel a stab in my heart. It feels like I can never believe in anything anymore. My mom was the strongest of all women. When I was growing up there was never anything she couldn't fix, not a hurt she couldn't touch and make better. What is this cosmic debacle that sentenced her to this debilitating, humiliating experience?

Tears slip down my face. I sniffle and look around for a tissue. I'm not really crying for myself. I'm crying for all those memories I have of my mother's arms outstretched, pushing me on a swing. Or for the times her arms would reach around to hold me and my brother or tickle us till we lay helpless on the floor. I can see her hands, strong and capable, making a home for us… cooking, feeding, nurturing. She and I have both changed, I guess. Now I am the one holding out my arms so she won't fall when she tries to get out of bed.

I think of the last time I was in this country, when I was graduating from high school. I was so carefree and young. I rushed everywhere on my bike, giddy with impending freedom, thinking it would last forever. I walked out of the school with the rest of my class, proudly wearing our white hats that showed that we had passed "studenten," the exam that sprang us from high school. I saw my mom in the crowd as we stood there having pictures taken and accepting congratulations. She was smiling, her eyes filled with happy tears.

Handing me a huge bouquet of spring flowers, she held me for a moment, cupped my cheek and said, "I'm so proud of you, my darling. I'm so proud of you."

Today I walked my mother to the room where she was to receive chemotherapy. I had so many emotions churning inside me that I couldn't distinguish one from the other. I still can't. I am torn between anger and sadness and pain.

My mom's hand shone, almost translucent against my brown skin as she leaned heavily on me. Just before she walked into the room, to be filled with chemicals that make her want to die, she looked back at me for a brief moment, smiled and winked at me. As I turned away to get my coffee and wait for her, I whispered:

"I'm proud of you, Mom. I'm so proud of you."

The author was born and raised in Sri Lanka where her Sinhalese father and Swedish mother ran an orphanage, hospital and community development project in the central hill country. She pursued her education in Sweden and in the United States. She has a deep interest in social work and third world development and has volunteered at relief projects in Romania and Sri Lanka as well as community-based relief projects in Sweden and the United States. Her work will be published in the anthologies *An Elephant in the Playroom* and *Special Gifts*, to be released in 2007. She is currently at work on a book of short stories.

Continued from page 124

Chemotherapy and Fertility

Chemotherapy can affect a woman's fertility by damaging the ovaries. The older a patient is at the time she begins chemotherapy, the more likely she is to suffer infertility. Chemotherapy can also produce an earlier menopause even if it does not make a woman completely infertile at the time of treatment, because it can reduce the number of functioning eggs. There are treatments available for women who wish to preserve their fertility and the science behind the various treatments is continuing to improve. Currently, the best method of preserving fertility is to freeze embryos. This involves in vitro fertilization, high dose hormones, and donor sperm from a husband, partner, or sperm bank. Hormones used in the treatment often include estrogen, which theoretically could be a problem if a patient has an estrogen receptor positive tumor; however, many oncologists feel one round of high dose estrogen may not pose an unacceptable risk to the patient. There are also drugs that can be used that are known to be safe in treating breast cancer, such as tamoxifen or letrozole. The options should be discussed with your doctor in advance, if possible.

Other possible options that are less well studied include *egg freezing*, where eggs are frozen without first being fertilized. Another, *ovarian tissue freezing* for later reimplantation, is less well studied. Still another is *gonadotropin-releasing hormone analog treatment*, a drug that can be given to suppress the activity of the ovaries and put them in a dormant state while the patient receives chemotherapy. Its effectiveness is currently under study.

Continued on page 162

Stage III, Act One

Mike Gowen

Breathe, Michael.

I remember reminding myself to breathe... just breathe. I sat in the waiting room with my family, well, waiting. It could have been minutes or hours, I really couldn't tell you. I just remember reminding myself to breathe, and the fear, unlike any I had known in my life.

We were waiting on biopsy results from a tissue sample taken from my mom's right breast. That sounds very matter of fact, as if we were waiting on a sandwich order. I don't mean to come across that way.

Mom had found a lump earlier in the year but had kept it to herself. Perhaps she thought it was nothing; she may have thought it would just go away. She may have thought she was protecting us. Like many before her, maybe she didn't want to know. Finally, she confided in her sister, who had the good sense to ignore Mom's demands for confidentiality and immediately called my dad. Mom was angry with my aunt for telling us. But that breach of confidence ultimately saved her life.

I remember the surgeon entering the waiting room carrying a handful of reports that would confirm our worst fear. Mom had breast cancer. It was Stage III, and it was metastatic. I was so shaken by the news that I felt ill. I looked over at my dad and for the very first time in my life, I saw him cry. That was the defining moment for me, the moment that made this tragedy real. Mom cried too, and she apologized for being sick.

I could fill page upon page with stories about my mom to help you understand what a remarkable woman she is. I'm not sure any of them reflects her capacity for love as much as her sitting in that doctor's office, having heard the most traumatic news of her life and apologizing to her family for it. Even at a time like this, Mom was thinking of everyone but herself. She was worried about what the family would be put through to take care of her. She was worried about the sacrifices others would have to make because she would be incapacitated, about who would be there for us if she died.

Me? I was worried about not passing out in front of my mom. I envy people who can cry when they want to. It doesn't come easy for me. I used to think it was just a man versus woman thing. Like somewhere along the way women got the gene for tears and men didn't. It could be that through gender ignorance I comprehend tears as a sign of weakness. Then again, it could be because I'm so logical in my thinking that by the time I figure out I should cry it's too late. I wish I had cried that day. I was angry with myself a long time because I didn't. Come to think of it, I still am.

To be honest, I've always regarded cancer as a death sentence. It's as if upon hearing the news you say, "Well, that's it then," and you proceed to make funeral arrangements. Fortunately, after extensive tests, we learned that Mom's cancer had only spread to the lymph nodes under her arm. Although the prognosis was still not good, we were elated with this news: it gave us hope that Mom could survive this deadly disease.

The next year was a blur of tests, waiting, treatment, more tests, and more waiting. It was the hardest thing I have ever been through. I can't imagine what it was like for Mom. Since her cancer was so advanced she was recommended an aggressive course of treatment that included a radical mastectomy of her right breast, removal of lymph nodes on her right side, chemotherapy and radiation. My mom, who never liked taking pills, was given drugs to help her rest, drugs to ease her anxiety, drugs to help with nausea brought on by treatments, and maintenance drugs to battle the cancer itself.

I used to think I was a patient person but cancer has a way of eating away at your patience. There are no quick fixes with cancer. We were always waiting. We waited for doctors, appointments, tests and test results. We waited for treatments to begin and treatments to end. I tried to be upbeat, to downplay disappointments in front of my mom. I was exhausted from not sleeping. I was frustrated and angry at the disease that had targeted her. I cursed God in one breath for allowing her to suffer and in the next I pleaded with Him for her life.

There is no way to sugarcoat the treatment process. It is ugly. And it hurt me so much to see her hurt. But today, Mom's cancer is in remission. Every few months she has blood tests and we wait anxiously for the results. As of this writing, she continues to be cancer free. Mom takes a maintenance drug daily to reduce the chance of the cancer returning. Mom's cancer evolved into a tremendous learning experience for our entire family, about the disease and about each other. We have always been a close family but this experience brought us even closer. We needed each other every day. We still need each other every day.

I pray for Mom to remain cancer free. Unfortunately, we don't get to choose. None of us do. I want to keep her with me as long as possible. I don't want her to undergo treatments again. If Mom's cancer does return, however, I will love and support her, be there for her and celebrate with her when she defeats it again.

Mike Gowen is a freelance writer living in Winston-Salem, North Carolina who has published numerous articles, many on parenting. He and his wife Anne have blended a family that includes six children and five grandchildren.

We Don't Dance Alone

Patricia McKenna

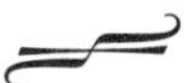

The hospital room was large and as warm and comforting as a hospital room can be. Complete with sofa, recliners, a table and chairs, it was a room designed for a family, with peaceful paintings and a large window overlooking the scenic Kankakee River. The only part of it that looked like a hospital was the bed in which my mom was lying.

My sister and I had been spending as much time with Mom as we could. As a matter of fact, all of Mom's kids agreed that she would never be alone during this hospital stay, so the four of us were taking turns spending the nights with her in that hospital room. This time, we didn't think she was going home.

"Do you need anything, Mom?" my sister asked.

"No," she replied, quickly adding, "Wait, yes I do." Mom continued, "Can you find out the names of those three nurses?"

"What nurses are you talking about?" we asked, somewhat confused. You see, Mom had one nurse assigned to her for each ten-hour shift, and we'd gotten to know them rather well in the past few days. Which was she referring to?

"Those three nurses who keep coming in here and standing at the foot of my bed," she replied. "They won't speak to me, and I want to know why."

Looking around, we didn't see any nurses, and then carefully but skeptically asked, "Are they here right now?"

Mom looked up, then she turned her head to look out the window. We were relieved when she replied that the nurses weren't there right then, but then she continued, "Look out the window. They're out there dancing on the river, but they'll be back in a few minutes. That's what they do. They stand here for a while and stare at me, and then they go out and dance on the river, and come back and stand here again. But they won't speak to me, and I think it's rude."

Spring had finally arrived in Illinois, and the river had thawed. Although we knew there were no nurses dancing on the river, my sister and I both walked to the window—just to be sure. As expected, the river was quiet and peaceful, without any dancing nurses.

Mom had talked to us about her cancer, but she never talked to us about dying. It was 1995, Mom was 54 years old, and she had fought the disease for eight years. In 1987, she had a mastectomy and tests showed that the cancer hadn't spread. We were all relieved that her physician had concluded that radiation and chemotherapy weren't necessary. But in 1993, Mom began having back problems. She saw a chiropractor, went to physical therapy, and even took a leave of absence at work because of the pain before anyone diagnosed the problem: the cancer had returned, this time metastasized to the bones.

Mom never told us that her disease was terminal. My sister and I found out during a private appointment with her new oncologist (it was years before the strict confidentiality laws had been enacted, and this doctor was very receptive to talking to patients' families, even going so far to say that he "treats the family as well as the patient").

"At this stage, 50 percent will live less than a year, and the other 50 percent may live a little more than a year," the doctor advised.

My sister and I listened quietly and then, softly, nervously, I asked, "Does she know this?"

"Yes," he solemnly replied. "It was the first question she asked me."

Speechless, we left his office. For three months now, Mom had known that she was in the last year of her life, and she hadn't said anything to us. Some people may think that's strange or even wonder if we were close to our mother. For Mom, it really wasn't that strange and yes, we were close. Mom was the best friend her two daughters had ever had, and we saw her almost every day and talked on the phone with her every night.

My mom was a warm yet strong person. Her strength had seen her through a divorce, a mastectomy and a hysterectomy, and aided her as she walked with her cancer-ridden back in her grandson's funeral procession. Now, she was undergoing radiation and chemotherapy treatments. Never once did she complain, always taking everything that life handed her and getting through each challenge one at a time. She wouldn't even take anything for pain, though there were often times we wished she would.

She was our rock, even when we should have been hers. We turned to her for comfort and support, never letting on that we knew her prognosis. We spent our days with her, talking about everything under the sun: our kids, music, careers and, inevitably, her favorite NASCAR driver, Ernie Irvan. Our time was spent learning everything we could about her and her childhood, how to cook our favorite dishes and enjoying the companionship of the woman we loved more than any other. Because Mom was calm, so were we. We followed her lead, respecting her decision not to share her prognosis with us. But we often wondered why she chose silence.

Looking back, I think I understand why. Even though her life was ending, she didn't want to spend her last year dying; she wanted to spend it living. She didn't want to spend her last year crying, and she didn't want her children to cry either. Mom got what she wanted: quality time with her children and grandchildren. Ultimately, it was what we wanted, too.

Mom's time with us exceeded her doctor's prognosis. She lived for almost two years after the fateful day she received her prognosis. Many times, we worried about how lonely it must have been for her to bear that knowledge alone. But now I know that she really wasn't alone. She shared her burden with her doctor, for whom she'd developed a great deal of respect and fondness. Her sisters and brothers who lived in Tennessee had visited several times. Her youngest brother was a minister, and she had confided in him, receiving spiritual and brotherly love and guidance to help her through.

As we sat in her hospital room three days before she lost her battle, Mom was still making sure that she was there for us, helping us accept the inevitable and letting us know that she wasn't alone. After all, she had us and the "three nurses" with her, whom she kept insisting were either in her room or on the river. Mom could see them clearly, although we couldn't see them at all. As her time drew nearer, though, we began to sense their presence, believing that they were patiently waiting to make sure she wasn't alone when she made her transition to the other side.

It was our mother's strength that helped us as we said goodbye, and it is her strength that we hold on to every day as we face life's challenges. And through it all, we remember that, like Mom, we're never really alone. Sometimes, when I need her the most, I look out at the river and believe that she's right there with me. Once in a while, I can even see her dancing.

A lifelong resident of Kankakee, Illinois, writer and editor Patti McKenna is a wife and mother of four daughters. Her diverse experience in the educational, health and legal fields lends itself to a wide variety of writing genres. Patti's gift for storytelling carries over into her songwriting career: she has had three songs published within the last year.

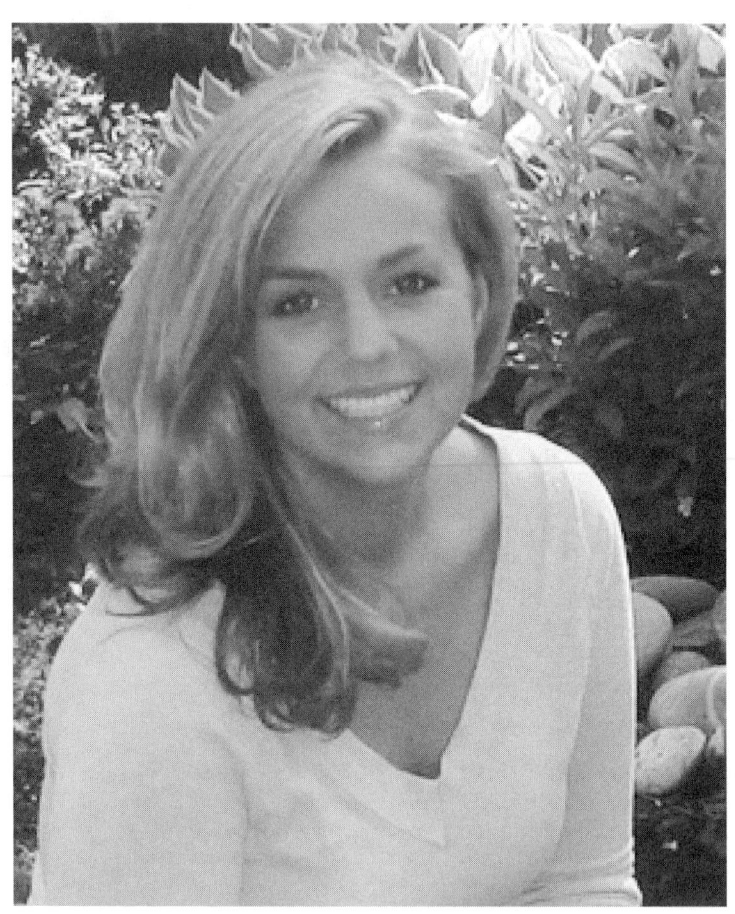

Emily Donohue Robbins

April Showers

Emily Donohue Robbins

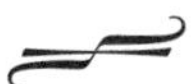

We stood together at the edge of the bathtub. My mother had just gotten home from the hospital this April day and her body was too weak to support itself. I lifted her right leg over the tub wall, then her left. She sat down on the folding plastic chair we had wedged into the tub, face lifted up to the water, eyes closed. She told me not to rush her, that she just wanted to sit and feel the water.

My terry-clothed hand rubbed her shoulder blades, around and around, giving birth to soap suds, propelled by the knowledge that it felt good to her. I massaged her scalp with shampoo, not missing one hair on her head. For the 53 years of her life, Patti Robbins loved to shower. She showered through the eight chemo-filled years of her breast cancer: her mastectomy; her multiple rounds of hair loss; her fatigue and vomiting; her radiation and brief remission; the cancer's metastasis to the anus and abdomen; her surgery to implant an external liver drain.

We hesitated when the palliative caregivers suggested that we take her home after several extended hospital stays. Our concerns dissolved when my mother told us that all she wanted to do was to take a shower at home, determined that the cancer would not rob her of her one indulgence. My father rush-ordered three types of shower seats, not knowing which would work best. Anxious to help, I skipped Senior Week celebrations at college, from which I would graduate in three weeks. Watching my mother close her eyes to the shower's tears that April morning, I knew how good it felt for her to rinse everything away.

We hadn't washed her butt; we would wait to do that at the end. When she was ready, I carefully soaped the lump around her anus and even more carefully rinsed the open sores around her vagina. I knew that my mother wanted to preserve her dignity, her privacy; I tried to ease her humiliation. "It's no biggie, Ma," I joked, "I've seen your butt before." When we were done I wrapped her shivering body in dryer-warmed towels.

My mother told me she liked it best when I helped her shower because I didn't rush her as much as everyone else did. I remember feeling then, at 22, like I'd won a prize by being able to give her something no one else could. I told her I had liked it best when she had bathed me as a child, that I'd especially loved it when she splashed in the water from the edge of the bathtub, shaping my soapsuds beard or my brother's mohawk, laughing until we washed away our soapy personas at the showerhead. During this April shower, I wished we were mermaids like we pretended to be when I was young, the bathroom filling with imaginary water, fish swimming gently by us.

After her bath I helped her climb the tub wall and she sat on the toilet to catch her breath. She bound her hair in a towel, twisted like soft serve ice cream. When I handed her the deodorant she lifted her arm, revealing the pea-sized, purple bumps down her side where the cancer had come through her pores. Her dexterity stolen by the neuropathy, she missed her armpit with the stick but I didn't say anything; it didn't matter. She let out an audible "*brrrrrr*" when I unwrapped the towels from around her shoulders. I quickly helped her on with an undershirt—bras didn't matter anymore. I guided her arms into a blue cardigan, the one whose fabric didn't irritate the skin on her arms, and chose socks to match her outfit, just as she always had during the years she had taught kindergarten.

She rested her head on my belly as I stood above her, rubbing her back to make warmth from the friction. I did not rub anywhere near her kidneys, where even the slightest touch hurt her. She exhaled heavily and touched the back of my knee with her right hand. I wished I had warmed more towels for her.

Edema had ballooned her ankles and weighed them down, so after she powdered between her legs, I lifted her left foot into her stretchy cotton pants, and then her right. After a deep breath we got her to her feet, pants up. There was a plastic chair next to the toilet, so she could sit again after dressing. She braced herself on my arms as I took baby steps backward and she followed, like I had followed her when I learned to walk. Careful not to brush the swollen lymph nodes under her arms as I lowered her—"I'm not a baby, you know," she breathed—I stepped away quickly, unsure of how to balance my wanting her to know just how much I had helped and allowing her to think she was still in control. I told her that of course she was not a baby, that I just wanted to help her.

I reached for the dangling bag into which emptied the bile that could no longer drain into her small intestine because a tumor pinched off the connecting duct. The bile stained bright yellow, spotting many of her white cotton nightgowns, so I was careful to hold the bag away from her. The stickiness of it glued the bag stopper shut and I could not twist off the cap. She tried and couldn't open it, either. We had to use pliers to pry open the tube, pointing it downwards into the container where we hoped bile would gush out, because the more bile that drained from her insides, the less leaked into her abdomen. "Two ounces," I told her, as I drained the bag—and we both knew it should have been four. I rinsed the rotten fish smell from the bag, then safety-pinned it to her underwear, a system my mother had invented to keep herself as mobile as possible. I encircled with sterile gauze the base of the tube entering my mother's abdomen. She reminded me to be careful, not to pull or twist, because she was sure her liver could be pulled out. I sealed around the tube with Tegaderm, trimmed neatly so as not to irritate more skin than was already angry with infection.

"Hand me the comb, will you?" she asked, eyes closing, fighting off the pain medication that made her so tired. She brushed her short curls backward, to the left. I asked if she wanted a mirror, she said no. "Do you want to wear earrings?" I asked, as I scanned the framed earring screen we'd painted two summers earlier. The novelty earrings—snowmen, breast cancer ribbons, ladybugs, angels—were surrounded by an array of colorful, stacked-bead earrings, sea glass, and tinted metals. We had made several of the earrings on vacation together. She organized her beads by color and guaranteed we would make a fortune from jewelry making. "How about these?" I asked, taking down her favorite pair, purple and green batik cardboard, and holding them up to her ears. "Only if it's not a hassle," she replied. I had never known her to refuse a pair of earrings; she'd always felt naked without them.

"Let's go sit together, what do you say?" I asked. I ran my fingers through her hair and helped her to her feet, guiding her slowly to the recliner that didn't hurt to sit in. She lowered herself and fell backwards, exhausted. I put her feet up and surrounded her neck with a U-shaped pillow so her head wouldn't loll from side to side. I put the pediatric-sized cannula under her nose so it would breathe oxygen into her tired body. I tucked an unruly curl behind her ear and covered her with two blankets so her cool cleanliness would not chill her.

"You smell so good," I told her after her eyes closed. Something in her throat rose and lowered. She didn't need to say a word to let me to know she was saying thank you.

For months after she died, I thought taking a shower would summon the intimacy of that last vivid memory, but I often felt only sorrow. I would picture her blemished body and wish that I could make more bubbles on her back, soothing her, touching the body in which she was captive, knowing she would have done the same for me.

Sometimes, after I have soaped my body, I sit on the shower floor, curled against the wall, water hot, and cry for my mother. I watch the rivulets of water swirl before they are lost to the darkness of the drain. There is security in the masked sobbing, and the moment is always naked. I have started to use a washcloth, not a loofa, as a small tribute to my mother. I often douse myself in her body spray, reliving her clean smell. These daily ritual changes help me remember how much my mother loved the water, drank the warmth, and how important it is to remember her loving. They help me know that it's okay to have memories so vivid that they hurt, but that I must also remember the memories so vivid that they make me laugh, like the time after a shower she told me to touch her wispy hair because it felt just like "duck fluff."

Now, when I think of the muscles in my mother's neck straining to enjoy her last shower, I think of the peace in her expression: eyes closed, lips drawn, her body capturing the warmth from the water. I think of the time just after her mastectomy that I gave her the black and white poster depicting a young girl who cupped her hands to catch the rain, smiling among her wet curls, captioned "Just as it seems it will never rain again, life comes back."

Emily Robbins grew up in New Hampshire, where she now works at the Center for Environmental Health Sciences at Dartmouth College. Her mother's eight-year struggle with breast cancer sparked her interest in community health, a subject in which she received a Bachelor of Arts degree from Brown University just four days before her mother died. Emily devotes much of her time to writing about her experiences with her mother's disease and other people's experience with illness; she believes that readers can find courage and inspiration from the stories of others.

Continued from page 146

Choosing a Surgeon

Traditionally, surgical breast care has been provided by the general surgeon. While most or many general surgeons still treat breast patients in their practices, over the last 20 years or so breast surgery has become established as a separate subspecialty, especially in large cities. The reasons for this are many. Issues surrounding breast care are very emotional and require an abundance of time and discussion. As the vast amount of research in the field has led to subtle changes in management and treatment and the surgeon needs to stay informed and educated. This requires a large amount of time and effort and a true dedication to the field. You will want a surgeon who is not only knowledgeable and technically skillful, but also someone who can explain clearly the type of treatment you will need and guide you through potential pitfalls along the way. If possible, seek the recommendation of a physician you trust. Also, remember that this will be a relationship that goes on for years after your surgery, so you must actually *like* the surgeon you choose, as you will be seeing a lot of him or her in the future. Make sure your surgeon takes the time you need to answer questions and explain procedures, doesn't try to rush you into decisions, and doesn't get annoyed should you ask if a second opinion might be beneficial (whether you get one or not). In any case, take the time you require to make an informed, well-thought-out decision about where to have your surgery.

Continued on page 170

Choices

Patricia F. D'Ascoli

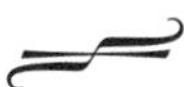

Breast self-exams were not something my mother and I discussed. I had never been very good at doing them and I had no idea whether my mother even did them. So I was a bit surprised one morning when she casually mentioned to me that she thought she had a lump in her breast. "What does it feel like?" I asked. "Kind of like a marble," she answered. Not good, I thought.

Our fears were confirmed a few days later when the gynecologist called the lump "suspicious" and recommended a biopsy. I trusted this man implicitly. He had seen me through three miscarriages, two successful pregnancies and a tubal ligation. He would never use that word unless he had a strong sense that the lump was abnormal.

Cancer. The word struck such fear into my heart. The disease killed both my stepfather and my sister. At 78, Mom had osteoporosis and congestive heart disease, and in the past few years had suffered several bouts of pneumonia. But breast cancer was something I had never thought about my mother having.

Mom accepted the news with aplomb. To her, nothing could be as bad as the severe depression she had experienced all her life as a result of bipolar disorder. To her, unlike depression, cancer could be cut out, possibly even cured. If Mom's mental state was up, as it most decidedly was when she was diagnosed, she felt her cancer was conquerable.

The surgeon offered Mom two choices. She could have either the entire breast removed (a mastectomy) or just the tumor and surrounding tissue (a lumpectomy.) Because the latter could not assure a complete elimination of the offending cells, if she chose a lumpectomy she would need to have radiation treatments. In all likelihood, she would also need to take tamoxifen, a drug which slows or stops the growth of breast cancer cells that are already present in the body.

I was surprised when my mother decided on a lumpectomy. Would it not be simpler and easier to have a mastectomy? I wondered why, at this late stage in her life, she would care about her appearance. But who was I to question whether any woman should willingly give up a breast when there were other alternatives available? Perhaps I might make the very same decision one day.

The surgery went well, according to the surgeon. His job was done; my mother's had just begun. Fortunately, the cancer had not spread. The radiation would finish off any lingering cancer cells. So far, so good, we thought, until we met with the oncologist, who informed us that my mother's breast cancer was not the "hormonal" type. Tamoxifen was no longer a possibility. Instead, she would need chemotherapy as well as radiation.

Visions of nausea, vomiting, hair loss and other nightmares entered my mind. Don't worry, the doctor told us. It's a low dose, so there shouldn't be any complications. But suddenly, everything was a complication. What would chemotherapy do to my mother's frail body? How sick would she become in an effort to fight a disease that could have been eradicated if only she hadn't been so vain? I kept these negative thoughts to myself as we sat in the oncologist's office, absorbing the news. She would need six doses of the cancer-destroying medication followed by a series of radiation treatments. None of this information seemed to faze my mother in the least.

We were grateful that our local hospital had a state-of-the-art cancer center with comfortable reclining chairs for patients to sit in while receiving chemotherapy. The nurses were wonderful, kind people, as was all the staff. The center ran like a well-oiled machine. But all its efficiency could not disguise the fact that war was being waged there.

Chemotherapy destroys good cells along with the bad, and this meant that my mother, who was prone to bronchial infections, would be at risk with a weakened immune system. After two or three chemotherapy sessions, she did indeed come down with a bronchial infection that turned into a serious case of pneumonia. She required hospitalization and aggressive antibiotic treatments. But Mom rallied, recovered from the pneumonia and continued on with the prescribed course of chemotherapy.

That February I celebrated my 40th birthday with my family. Mom, who was feeling well both mentally and physically, joined us for dinner and enjoyed a nice meal with a little champagne and some birthday cake. She had just one more treatment session and would then begin radiation. It really looked like my mother was going to beat this cancer.

Apparently Mom's body had other plans for her. Early one morning soon after the party, she collapsed. Her left leg had suddenly given way. Stranded at home with three young children on a snowy morning, I called an ambulance and waited next to my mother on the floor, trying to comfort her until it arrived. Mom's femur had completely shattered, requiring a lengthy operation to repair the bone. After her hospital stay she was transferred to a rehabilitation center for three months of physical therapy. The dreaded depression returned, clouding her tenuous recovery with insecurity and the fear that she would never walk again.

Yet somehow, perhaps with the promise of a warm spring on the horizon, Mom's strength and resolve improved and she came home, having finally mastered the use of a walker. The oncologist told us that, although she had not completed all of the chemotherapy sessions, she'd had enough to allow her to go ahead with the radiation.

How much more could my mother possibly endure? Even though I knew that this final phase was necessary, I just wanted Mom to be done with it all. Now she would have to go to the cancer center every weekday for five weeks, a beam of powerful radiation directed at a targeted area on her breast. What further havoc would this wreak on her frail system?

Mom faithfully attended all of the radiation sessions and we were assured of a positive outcome. The survival rates were good for patients who had experienced the kind of breast cancer Mom had. Free at last from her cancer center commitments, Mom and I looked forward to a healthy summer which would include a family vacation in California. It was the last trip she would ever take.

In the months preceding her death, Mom's immune system grew steadily weaker. The doctors were ultimately unable to treat or even name the disease process that had taken over. I knew in my heart that it was a result of the chemotherapy, something that could have been avoided had she decided upon a mastectomy.

But there was little sense in blaming something my mother had willingly chosen to do. Her choices may not have been what I wanted, but they were, in the end, hers alone to make. Fiercely determined to win, she fought cancer in her own way.

Patricia D'Ascoli is a freelance journalist who writes for newspapers and magazines. She also publishes a literary newsletter, *Connecticut Muse*, and is the author of *Home Is Where the Humor Is*, a collection of essays about family life. She lives in Connecticut with her husband and their three sons.

A Breast Cancer Epic...
for my sister
Deborah L. Bohlmann

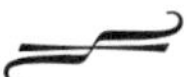

You know me as Odysseia,
survivor of journeys
fraught with monsters,
as one cursed and released
by the gods of breast cancer.
Now I do them obeisance,
walking inland with oar
on my shoulder,
awaiting the land dweller's call.
Tell us your tale,
they demand from the fields,
your story of bravery and woe.
Tell of outsmarting
the brutal Cyclops of surgery,
oozing green lymph from a tube in your armpit,
carrying scars of battle survived
onward and further forever.

Tell how you faced the vicious six-headed dog-creature
of chemotherapy,
each treatment a blow in itself,

each week another pull of the oars toward health,
along the way sacrificing the companionship of
energy and beauty and comfort,
driven by the strength
of fellow adventurers.

Tell how you endured the relentless whirlpool
of radiation,
each day another rotation
of buzzing, burning rays,
chewing up the skin,
chests tattooed in alien color,
held aloft by the branches of kindness
among technicians and nurses
who dare reach out over these monstrosities,
shelter and prophet at once.

The good doctor Athene,
goddess of war and wisdom and oncology,
renders swift advice,
appears with each conflict,
foresees the troubles and the victories.

At home, my own Penelope, my husband
waits up long nights,
weaving blankets of hope
on looms without end.
I am missing,
gone to war far away,
my return a promise
unfinished.
He endures with a memory of me,
never resting
while our bed awaits,
once a living tree,
the cornerstone of home.

My children, my dear Telemachi,
employ their newest bravery.
Into the world they venture,
carrying their lost mother before them,
pink wristband for a sword,
youthful energies applied to seeking a way
on their own.
They grow up without me
while I fight my distant monsters,
but they remain true to me,
molded by their father's presence,
hearkening to who we were together once,
traveling on in confidence
of who we will be again.
Divine eyes watch over them.

So now I've come home,
the hall clearing at last
of those unruly suitors,
medication and pain.

I stride on,
my oar over my shoulder.
Yes, I answer those
who have never ventured to the shore,
never traveled the infinite open waters
in a simple wooden boat.
Yes, I am the one you have heard of,
who survived monsters unthinkable,
who fought her way home.

Deborah L. Bohlmann is a mother to three teens. A breast cancer survivor, she enjoyed a 25-year career teaching high school English.

Continued from page 162

Getting a Second Opinion

Because there are often many choices of treatment for breast cancer, many people get second opinions. Does everyone need a second opinion? The answer is no. If you are comfortable with your surgeon, medical oncologist and radiation oncologist, you received your referral from a reliable source and you are completely satisfied with the treatment plan, do not feel obligated to get a second opinion. However, there are many times when it might be helpful. Breast cancer is a complicated subject and sometimes hearing the information more than once and in a slightly different way is helpful in understanding your condition. If you are told you need a mastectomy but are not convinced that this is the right course of action, seek a second—and perhaps a third—opinion. If you are given several different choices of chemotherapies to consider and you are not sure how to proceed, get another opinion. However, do not simply keep looking for the doctor who is willing to tell you what you want to hear just to get you in their door. It is most important to do lots of research before your doctor visit and when a physician gives you an opinion, make sure it is a well-thought-out plan by asking questions.

Continued on page 186

Part V

I AM TAKING CHARGE

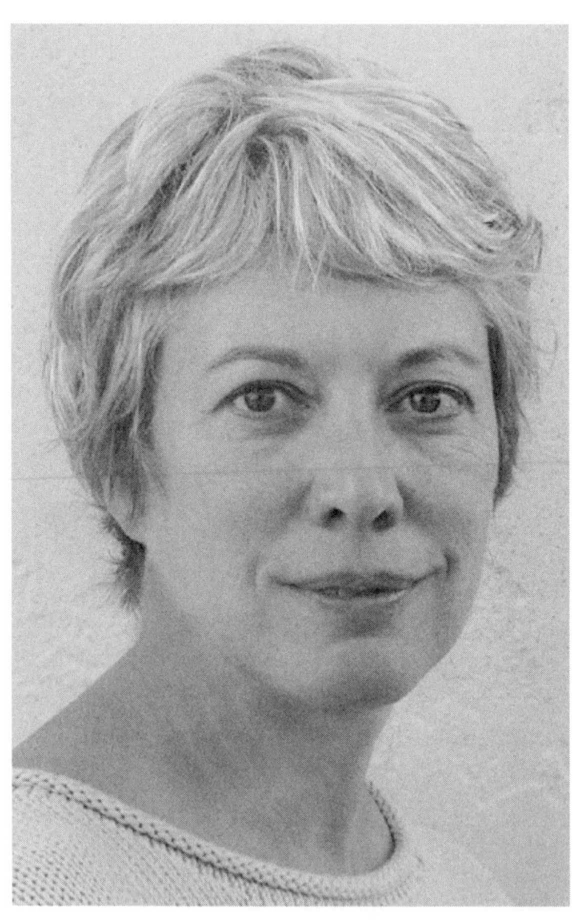

Deni Elliott

Whose Cancer Is It Anyway?

Deni Elliott

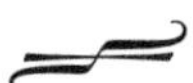

The oncology nurse and I played telephone tag Monday and Tuesday. She wouldn't sound so chipper if there were anything wrong, I told myself.

We finally connected on Wednesday, and that's when I learned I had breast cancer. The nurse reached me five minutes before a meeting at the agency where I am the ethics officer. I told the nurse I understood what she was telling me. I said I would call back in half an hour.

I assume that I walked down the hall to my meeting. I remember none of what happened once I got there, nor what happened that day, aside from telling my husband, telling my mother, telling my staff.

I soon learned that the surgeon had had the diagnosis in hand the previous Friday, but had left for a conference without sharing it with me. Inadvertently, he left me worried and wondering while the nurse and I missed connecting. Later, he said that he didn't call me on Friday because he "didn't want to ruin my weekend." I thought I deserved to hear the news immediately from the doctor who could answer my questions rather than later from the nurse who deflected them. That's why I fired my first surgeon.

Now, here's why I fired my first oncologist...

I spent the week between my diagnosis and my first meeting with the oncologist who was to oversee my treatment surfing the Internet, absorbing all that I could about "locally advanced breast cancer." I stayed desperately intellectual, focused on climbing the steepest learning curve of my life. When I met the doctor, I opened a single-spaced typed page, organized by subcategories: *further diagnosis*, *treatment*, and *beyond*. She calmly listened past my mispronunciations as I asked my first question. Her response overflowed with unfamiliar terms like "cytology" and "differentiation." I tried my second question. I scribbled down what she said: "FISH," "HER2Neu," "ER/PR."

I shook my head. "I don't understand these terms without definitions. I don't have a medical degree."

"That's why you just have to trust us," she said.

I disagreed. I moved from one award-winning breast cancer research center to the next in my semi-successful attempt to find medical personnel willing to guide me through this involuntary adventure in language I could understand.

Never have I felt so vulnerable. Worse than the cancer was feeling incapable of breaking the code that would let me understand the information about my condition. Every medical practitioner shared my goal of helping me survive. But there the shared agenda ended. The medical system was constructed in such a way that I was to be a passive object of care. I insisted on being an active partner.

From the beginning, I was at odds with medical conventions. I approached cancer as if I had been taking a tax issue to an accountant or a legal issue to a lawyer. I did my best to hire a team of fiduciaries for my cancer care. But few doctors were ready for my approach. And support staff's priority seemed to be protecting doctors from their patients rather than supporting the professional relationship between fiduciary and client. I found the medical world to be one of function and biology filled with strangers who called me sweetheart and who expected me to simply present my body to them for procedures and treatment.

I ultimately chose my treatment center based on its philosophy of a multidisciplinary approach and including the patients as part of the decision-making team. During my initial six-hour appointment, my slides and I had attention from physician-researchers, residents and fellows. In between, volunteers who were "living with cancer" stopped in with coffee and conversation. The social worker pronounced me "information-seeking" and "appropriately anxious." The medical oncologist who happened to be on duty for multi-team review was the one assigned to be my primary doctor, but their team approach meant that I would have the expertise of the whole group of researcher-clinicians. With my input, it was decided that I would have four months of chemotherapy prior to a double mastectomy, then radiation and hormonal therapy. Due to my prior professional commitments, treatment was scheduled to begin in three weeks. I left thinking that I had found cancer nirvana. I didn't know that this was the last day that I would be included in multidisciplinary team meetings or in any conversation at all.

The next day, I realized I had questions: Which chemo would I get? What about nausea control? Could I take Neulasta and Aranisp immediately or did I have to wait until my blood counts went to hell? My treatment center was more than an hour's drive from home. What should I do in an emergency?

I called the oncologist to whom I had been assigned. Voicemail instructed that if this was a life-threatening emergency, hang up and dial 911. Press 1 for doctor appointments, 2 for chemotherapy appointments, 3 for medical records and so on until option 8: record a message for my doctor. So I left a message. It was ignored.

I tried once each day, pushing random numbers until, Day 4, I reached a live human. The doctor was out of town, but Phone Person said she'd leave her a message.

I called again the next week, apologizing for being a pest, but hoping to talk to the doctor. The doctor is very busy as she is just back in town, Phone Person said, but she'd leave a message. I called daily, left messages, and waited for the phone to ring. By now, my anxiety was more than appropriate, but I couldn't get the social worker to call me back to confirm that fact.

Finally, three days before treatment was to begin, Phone Person said that the doctor would not speak to me until I came in for my treatment.

The doctor would not speak to me. I had to repeat that sentence before it sank in. I wasn't prepared for this. The doctor would not speak to me? I looked at the list of questions that I wanted answered before my first chemo. I tried not to panic, tried to be creative. I sent a fax: "Dear Doctor, I understand that you are not willing to speak to me prior to our appointment, when I will begin my chemotherapy. Unfortunately, I have questions that I think need to be addressed before I start treatment. I apologize for the intrusion." I reduced my list to the three most urgent questions. And I waited some more.

An office assistant called me back a day before my treatment was to begin. The doctor said, she informed me, "We'll discuss all of this when I see you."

When I saw her, the doctor was warm, caring and responsive. She seemed unperturbed when I told her about my frustrating attempts to get information that would help me prepare for this journey. But I was indeed frustrated. In fact, whenever I walked into that office for a doctor's appointment, a chemo infusion, or a shot of Neulasta, I waited at least 30 minutes—even when I called ahead to confirm that I would be seen on time. I couldn't help but feel that I waited simply because someone decided that I would wait.

And the waiting wasn't the only thing that was frustrating. As someone with expertise in research ethics, I thought I understood all about informed consent. Theoretically, patients have the right and the responsibility to choose their clinical options. Ideally, they review the risks and benefits and alternatives and then make their treatment choices. But there was not one time in my cancer treatment year that giving consent approached this ideal. I found that when I was asked to give "consent," I was actually signing forms to protect the doctors and hospitals from liability and allowing information to be released to my insurance company. The forms called "consent" asked me to agree to go to arbitration rather than jury trial in case something went wrong. The consent forms let me know that whatever I was about to have done included some rare but unfortunate side effects including death. It's been the same with all the consent forms since then. Rarely has one included a description of the actual procedure. Never have they included alternatives.

Toward the end of the year, my doctor scheduled me for a bone scan. When I reviewed the consent form the day of the procedure, I noticed that I was consenting to be photographed for scientific or educational purposes, consenting to pay the bill, and consenting to a generic list of medical and surgical procedures that were generally unrelated to this procedure. I asked the receptionist what would happen if I didn't sign.

"Then we don't do it," she said.

"I've never had a bone scan," I said. "Is there something that explains what I'm agreeing to have done?"

The receptionist chewed her gum thoughtfully. "No. But you can ask Bobby when he gives you your shot."

"Oh, I'm going to get a shot," I said. "Can you tell me why?"

"Nope. Bobby can tell you."

I signed the form and waited for Bobby.

When Bobby came to inject me with radionuclide, he had no explanation of the procedure, nor could he explain what he was injecting me with aside from saying, "It's just some dye. I keep telling them that they should have brochures for the patients."

The most ludicrous instance of my giving consent was when I was least competent to do so. I lay in the recovery room after the mastectomy and reconstructive surgery, hazily realizing that it was over. Suddenly, activity. "Her blood pressure is 70," said one voice. "Crit's at 15," said another. "Get some blood in here NOW!" said a third.

"This isn't good," I thought.

Then my plastic surgeon stood over me. "You've developed some internal bleeding and we're taking you back to surgery."

It occurred to me that this might be serious when my mother and husband were ushered into the recovery room. Just then, someone waved a clipboard in front of me and said, "Hurry up. You need to sign the consent form."

Consent? I couldn't remember my name at that point or locate my hand to pick up a pen.

"My husband," I mumbled, I think. Though he remembers signing something, he certainly doesn't know what he signed.

This is not consent. It is waiver of liability. It is fine for patients to sign waivers, but shouldn't the documents be labeled correctly? I was amazed to find that the American Medical Association provides a description of informed consent close to what I thought it was before my cancer year. "Informed consent," the AMA says, "is more than simply getting a patient to sign a written consent form. It is a process of communication between a patient and physician that results in the patient's authorization or agreement to undergo a specific medical intervention." The goal of that communication, which includes solicitation of patient questions, is for the patient to be able to make an "informed decision to proceed or to refuse a particular course of medical intervention." There clearly is a divide between theory and practice.

Medical professionals create obstacles to optimum care when they fail to empower their patients by including them in the process. In this day of rapidly evolving research data, cancer treatment is a series of best guesses learned from some patients who have come before. But, each presenting individual has her own needs and own risk tolerance, along with her own unique set of errant cells. Failure to empower the patient eliminates the primary decision-maker from the choices that need to be made in her own care.

I had to empower myself. I became determined to be my own advocate. Because of that, my treatment was different from what it otherwise would have been: I had chemotherapy before surgery, with the result that I have the troubling, but important, knowledge that the drugs achieved only a partial remission. I had a double mastectomy, because I didn't want to risk the "slightly" abnormal cells in my left breast becoming cancerous as well.

I had immediate reconstruction because I was determined that my body image not be collateral damage in the "war" on my cancer.

I got more aggressive radiation therapy than the radiation oncologist had planned because I was educated by researchers about what counted as "optimal therapy." I have argued successfully to be treated as though I've had a recurrence with the hope that such aggressive treatment will prevent one.

No one can predict if I will die from cancer, or die with it, or one day be called "cancer free." But, if I do face recurrence, it is with certainty that everything that could have been done to prevent it was done. My treatment reflects last week's research findings, not "standard of care."

There is more than one answer to each of the questions that arise with diagnosis. While medical personnel should present all alternatives, they rarely do. Fiduciaries, consent, and empowerment are essential elements of being engaged with one's own treatment, but are largely absent from the current medical model.

Deni Elliott holds the Poynter Jamison Chair in Media Ethics and Press Policy at University of South Florida, St. Petersburg and serves as Ethics Officer for the Metropolitan Water District of Southern California. Deni is the author, co-author or editor of seven books, three documentaries, and more than 100 articles and book chapters for the lay, trade and scholarly press. Her co-hosted radio show, *Ethically Speaking*, aired in public radio markets 2002–2006. A new book in progress, *An Involuntary Adventure*, co-authored with her husband, Paul Martin Lester, explores the ethical and social justice implications of breast cancer diagnosis and treatment.

Re-Imaging

Mary Armao McCarthy

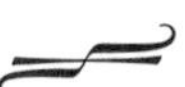

The customer service representative sounded embarrassed as she told me that my health insurance would pay for only one breast prosthesis. She hesitated, then went on, "for the rest of your life." I tried not to dwell on what seemed to be the company's expectation that I would not last long enough to need a replacement. Since my diagnosis with breast cancer, I had alternated between fear so strong it made my teeth chatter and an almost out-of-body composure as I obtained information, took notes and conducted the research project of my life.

It was hard to accept that I was in the subset of women for whom a lumpectomy was not an option. I found myself thinking back to a spring morning almost twenty years earlier, when an older neighbor, Mrs. Grazier, called to me from her side door. When I walked over, she reached down, took me by the arm, swooped me up the steps into her kitchen and pressed my hand to her breast. I was so startled that her excitement and happiness registered before her words took hold. Then it dawned on me: she was telling me she had recently had reconstructive surgery after her mastectomy. She'd had to fight for it. Insurance companies then wouldn't cover it, calling the procedure cosmetic. But finally, a victory: she was able to have a breast implant, paid for through her veteran's benefits from her service in the Women's Army Corps during World War II. Years later, I took special note of a court ruling on gender discrimination that gave all women the same victory. At least this was one problem I would not face now. Or so I thought.

I ordered the prosthesis so I would have it when I came home from the hospital. Breast reconstruction would take place later. I prayed I would have the courage to meet the challenges ahead, to make the best decisions, to survive surgery and chemotherapy, and to face an altered body. After my mastectomy, I was flat on one side, a C-cup on the other. Knowing that I could have breast reconstruction helped me to deal with this part of my disease. My mastectomy was clinically curative and breast reconstruction was emotionally healing.

My surgeries and treatments were arduous, but thankfully by the following year my cancer was in remission. I was pleased with the reconstruction. While it is not every woman's choice, I found it eliminated the constant reminder of my cancer when I dressed, lounged in my bathrobe with my kids and during intimate moments with my husband.

But then my implant shifted, moving higher on my chest. It hurt. It looked lumpy. I became the queen of vests. I saw my doctor. Yes, this just happens sometimes, she told me. A corrective procedure was scheduled. And then I got an unexpected call from my surgeon. She said my HMO had denied coverage for my surgery. They considered it to be cosmetic. I was stunned. Cosmetic? I thought women had won this battle. My insurer advised that if I were in more pain, they might have granted approval. More pain? How much pain did they want? I didn't think that there should have to be any pain at all.

Convinced this wasn't possible, that this couldn't happen to women any more, I called my insurance company. My doctor provided the additional information they requested. Two days before my surgery date, my doctor phoned me again. The insurance company had conducted an additional review of my case and they would still deny the surgery. My doctor was going to cancel the operating room.

I asked her to wait. I walked to a corner of my office where others could not see me and quietly wept. No one wants to have an operation. To fight for one is gruesome and harrowing. Struggling to compose myself, I went to the phone. Because I worked for a medical association, I could make calls to colleagues who handled health issues for the state legislature. They made calls. I learned later that my friends had not only gone to bat for me, they had gone straight to the top. The Governor's office and the leadership of both houses of the New York State legislature contacted my insurance company. The next day, as I worked at my desk, my HMO called. My surgery was approved. So sorry, they said, it had all been a mistake.

I was pleased for myself but outraged for other women. For others, this "mistake" would have stood. When I returned to work after a successful operation, I began speaking with patient and physician groups. I learned that women who had undergone lumpectomies as well as mastectomies were being denied breast reconstruction at all stages and the denials were increasing rapidly. Women were again suffering this injustice.

I am a private person, and I had not expected to discuss my cancer publicly. But I reached out, and the same colleagues who had helped win my insurance approval now joined with me to work for broader reforms. Lawmakers, medical groups and patient advocates collaborated. A large, multi-group press conference was organized at Memorial Sloan-Kettering Cancer Center in New York City. I was one of the final speakers, and as I began, I realized that most people had assumed I was there solely to provide a statement of support from my office, the American College of Obstetricians and Gynecologists. As I shared my personal story as well, the room grew ever more quiet. I finished to total silence. And then came an outpouring of support.

Legislation was introduced in New York State and nationally. The support of federal and state legislators was strong. I testified before the United States Senate and presented information at state and national forums. Women with breast cancer and legislators stood together at press conferences to seek reform. And we regained the victory women deserve. By the landmark legislation, comprehensive federal and state laws now require insurance coverage at all levels for women with breast cancer who choose breast reconstruction.

Today, women need to be aware of their rights. Instances of denials for breast reconstruction are infrequent now, but they do happen. Women and physicians need to know the law and pursue approval if needed. Not all women select reconstructive surgery, as is appropriate and as is their choice. But for women who want breast reconstruction after a mastectomy or lumpectomy, the option is there.

My health insurance company has changed its policy now and provides more than one breast prosthesis, authorizing a replacement at regular intervals. As is now required by law, they provide full breast reconstruction for cancer patients. Occasionally, a woman with breast cancer still contacts me for information. One, Diana, recently had reconstruction after a mastectomy ten years earlier. She reached me afterwards to say she was happy and felt like her old self. "And my doctor and I have a message for you," she added. "*Thanks.*"

Mary Armao McCarthy is the retired Executive Director of the American College of Obstetricians and Gynecologists, New York State. She was instrumental in the passage of legislation to secure insurance mandates for reconstructive surgery for women with breast cancer. Mary is a past Woman of the Year of the New York State Center for Women in

Government and Civil Society and the subject of a joint resolution of the New York State legislature honoring her work on women's issues. A past president of the Hudson Valley Writers Guild, Mary has published articles, essays and poetry and has been a contributor to northeastern public radio, but her favorite role is that of a mother and grandmother.

Continued from page 170

Breast Reconstruction

When breast conservation is not possible or a woman prefers to have a mastectomy, she may decide to reconstruct her breast. The first phase of reconstruction is usually done at the time of the mastectomy. There are two main forms of reconstruction. *Implants* are placed under the muscle of the chest wall. *Autologous tissue transfer* is a procedure where tissue is taken from another part of the patient's body and is used to reconstruct the breast. The most common areas from which tissue is taken are the abdomen (*transverse rectus abdominus muscle [TRAM] flap*), the back (*latissimus dorsi flap*), or the buttock (*gluteal flap*). There are many reasons why a patient may be a candidate for one form of reconstruction but not another. These issues need to be discussed both with your breast surgeon and your plastic surgeon. Many women have concerns about the cost of reconstruction. It is important to remember that if a mastectomy is covered by your insurance plan, then by law the reconstruction is covered as well, as long as you seek the care by a plastic surgeon in your health care network.

Continued on page 203

The Cure

Deborah Shouse

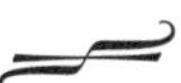

What would you do if someone said to you, Give me twenty-one days and I can help heal your cancer? I found out for myself.

"You have the best kind of breast cancer, quite contained," my doctor told me when I arrived at her office with my life partner, Ron. My hand shook as I wrote down the surgical treatment options. She told me I had six weeks before my surgery to prepare myself.

Later, after Ron drove me home I lay in bed, stunned and numb. How could this happen to me, Miss tofu-broccoli-vegetarian-exercise-meditation-prayer Shouse? How could I have breast cancer? I prayed, "Please help me understand the lessons in this. Please let me receive the healing I need." I fell asleep and when I awoke, I knew this illness was to be a spiritual journey.

Vowing to approach treatment with an open mind, I began reaching out, gathering advice and healing ideas. A friend recommended a medical intuitive. I had never personally encountered a medical intuitive, and I was curious. The intuitive asked me to send her a photo of myself and six pieces of my hair. A week later, she called and gave me a reading.

"Dear, darling," she said, "Don't let them cut you. I can help you heal in twenty-one days. Give me twenty-one days."

"Does this mean the lump in my breast will be gone?" I asked her.

"Yes."

"And if it is not?"

"I will help you prepare for surgery," she said.

I was intrigued by her offer. Part of me did not believe and part of me liked the fact that she was holding herself to a time limit. I scheduled my lumpectomy for a week after the twenty-one day period and began my healing journey.

Once I decided to go with the intuitive's regimen, I felt a sense of calm. I had a plan. At the end of the twenty-one days, I would have a sonogram and see if my lump had diminished or vanished. If so, hallelujah! If not, I would have the surgery.

During the next three weeks I gave up sugar, yeast, all prepared foods, fried foods, and more. I embraced a routine of supplements and homeopathy. I took herbal baths and rubbed my body with a cloth, proclaiming that I loved myself. I wrote in my journal and tried to release old hurts and fears. I prayed and meditated, used imagery to see my cancer cells dissolving and flooding out of my body. I let myself be cradled by the kindness and compassionate caring of my friends and family.

On the twenty-third day, Ron and I got on a plane to go meet with the intuitive. My hands were sweating when we stepped into the modern building that housed her office. When we met, she hugged me and I felt her warmth and compassion. She ushered me into a small room, intently scanned my body with her eyes and told me she felt the cancer cells were fifty percent gone. Another six weeks of diet and nutrition, she thought, and they might all be gone. I felt a rush of joy at the reduction and a stab of disappointment at the fifty percent still present. Still, I left her office feeling buoyant, certain I would see positive changes on the sonogram.

The night before the sonogram I prayed, "Please let me understand the results of the sonogram so I clearly know what to do next."

The sonogram was taken by the same person on the same machine as the earlier one. My lump showed no shrinkage.

The lump is the same, the same, played in my mind on the ride home. Disappointment welled inside me. I had hoped for concrete proof that my healing efforts had worked. As I slumped against my seat, Ron gently reminded me of last night's prayer: to clearly know what to do next. That prayer had been answered. I knew it was time for surgery.

"Healing takes many different forms," a friend quietly advised me. "Now it is time to surrender. It is time to let go of the notion of control and go into the flow."

I let the words sink into me. I remembered my initial prayer—that I receive the healing and lessons I needed. The healing work had helped me feel strong, powerful and purposeful in those confusing and scary early weeks. Following the intuitive's plan gave me time to research treatment options, gather information, shape my own healing ideas and hopes. During the six weeks between diagnosis and surgery, I felt flashes of nervousness and fear, but I never felt like a sick person: I felt vibrant and alive and full of promise.

In the days before surgery, my friends brought me food, prayer shawls, spiritual books, candles, soothing lotions and fuzzy socks. My spirit was opened, allowing me to truly feel and appreciate the outpouring of support, love and empathy.

I remembered advice I had read years ago: When you pray, make sure you are willing to see the answer to that prayer in whatever form it takes. I had prayed for healing. Though my lump had not disappeared in the way I had hoped, my prayers had been richly answered.

Deborah Shouse is a speaker, writer and editor. Her writing has appeared in *Reader's Digest*, *Newsweek*, and *Spirituality & Health*. She is donating all proceeds from her book *Love in the Land of Dementia: Finding Hope in the Caregiver's Journey* to Alzheimer's disease programs and research.

Lessons Learned

Tom Brown

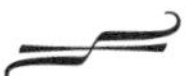

"The tumor is malignant." Those four words spoken by Dr. Don Colacchio in 1992 changed my life forever. The tumor was in the right breast of my wife, Barbara. She had inflammatory breast cancer, one of the rarest and most aggressive varieties. After the initial consultation with Barbara's oncologist, she and I sat down and developed a strategy of how we were going to deal with her disease. It was a simple plan: Barbara would be the patient and I would be the caregiver. We vowed to fight the disease and beat breast cancer.

I took our plan very seriously and followed it to the letter. As the caregiver, I did some things right and some things wrong. One right thing I did was to keep copious notes in a daily journal. I wrote down every detail of her treatment, including the type and amount of drugs that she took and the date and time she took them. I noted how she was feeling and documented any physical change, such as a spike in temperature, loss of appetite, nausea, pain or discomfort. There were several times during her treatment that the doctors needed the exact information I had in my journal. I would never have remembered all of it if I hadn't written it down.

Unfortunately, Barbara lost her battle in August of 1994, twenty-one months after her diagnosis. But we did all in our power to beat it. And I learned that being a caregiver means developing the ability to juggle many things every day. Yes, it was hard work, but it was worth it every step of the way. Here are a few of the most important lessons I learned.

Communication. This is probably the most important job and perhaps the most difficult to accomplish by the caregiver, particularly if the caregiver is a man. After diagnosis, the cancer patient will have to live with the physical, emotional and social consequences of having cancer. The caregiver must be able to listen to the needs of the patient effectively. Listen to her fears and be supportive. There are no magic answers. Be mindful that men and women generally communicate differently. Women often express their feelings more openly. When your loved one is talking, listen intently before offering a response. Sometimes she only wants you to hear how she feels and is asking for support, not advice. A simple hug and telling her "I understand, and will always be here for you," is all the response that is needed. She still needs to hear that you love her and always will.

Be mindful of the relationship you have developed with your loved one. If you were not good communicators before the cancer, don't expect to become great ones overnight; it might take some time. But both of you *must* make an effort to express your feelings. If you were good communicators, build on that relationship. This period in your life will be one of the most stressful you will ever endure, and the ability to understand each other is essential in order to get through it.

Finally, remember that there are other family members who must be included in what is happening. If there are children at home, keep them in the loop. Parents, siblings and friends are important too. They will want to know how the both of you are doing.

Be prepared for the pitfalls. There will be hurt feelings. You or the patient will say something that will be taken the wrong way. As the caregiver, you will try your best to give support and make sure the patient is comfortable. But you will be tired and stressed. The patient can mistake your tone of voice and be hurt by what you say. The patient too will be under constant stress. There will be times when she just does not know what to say. Tell her that it is okay. Offer up an alternative to talking about her feelings, such as writing them down in a daily journal.

Educate yourself. Most male caregivers have no idea what is involved in caring for a loved one who has breast cancer. It is imperative that the caregiver learn as much about the disease as possible as quickly as possible. There are hundreds of sites on the Internet devoted to the subject. The cancer treatment facility that you are using has useful brochures and pamphlets to help you better understand breast cancer.

You should learn as much as you can about the treatment your loved one will undergo. I suggest taking a tape recorder to every meeting with your doctors and ask for their permission to record the session. At the very least, you should keep your own journal with very detailed notes including the date, time, type and amount of drugs that your loved one is taking. There is a very good chance that she could develop an infection and have to be hospitalized. With your notes you can easily tell the attending physician what medication she has taken and when. You will have to be the one to educate the rest of your family and pass along the important information on your loved one's treatment. Try not to shield your loved one from your family and friends. Knowledge is power. The more that select family members know about the disease and treatment, the more they will be able to rally the kind of support that is needed. They will be able to anticipate when extra help or a meal or a visit is most needed.

Take care of yourself. Regardless of your age and physical condition, as a caregiver you will experience both emotional and physical stress. You will feel shock, anger, fear, sorrow, guilt, and maybe even hate, just to name a few. If you are a full-time employee, you will have to balance your work with taking care of your loved one. There are domestic responsibilities of tending the house, cooking, etc. If there are children at home, they need your attention also. Caregiving is demanding and stressful regardless what the circumstances are. Your journal, which can be as simple as a spiral notebook, isn't just a good place to keep track of the details of your loved one's treatment, but your own emotions as well. Take some time at the end of each day and jot down your feelings. It is a way of venting, and it is useful. And you must take care of your physical health. If you are not eating or sleeping properly, it will eventually affect your judgment and your health. If you get a cold or the flu and cannot care for your loved one, seek help from a family member or a friend. This backup caregiver should be involved from the beginning so they can step in at a moment's notice to make the transition. It would also be very helpful to find a friend or family member to look out for *your* well-being. Ask them to check on you daily, even if it is just a phone call to see how you are doing. You need it and deserve it.

Come to grips with reality. I have been a problem solver my entire life. I am not always successful and I make mistakes on occasion. But I enjoy a hard challenge and take great pleasure when I complete a task. The challenge of helping my wife beat cancer was a problem I never thought I would have to face. It just always seemed that since we were such a happily married couple, we would enjoy the golden years together. I had a very difficult time knowing that I couldn't do a thing to cure Barbara. All I could do was fight along with her and provide as much comfort and support as I could. During our journey, I did a lot of soul searching and philosophical pondering about the meaning of life in general. I found that I had a very hard time focusing on anything but the battle with cancer. It was all-consuming.

But I also found that I had strengths I didn't know I had. When you are at the lowest ebb in your life, somehow you can find the strength to carry on. I found that I was much more pleasant with people than I ever had been before. At the same time, I found myself wishing that someone else had my problems. I would see couples in perfect health and ask, "Why not them?" Not that I actually wanted them to have cancer, but I just wanted it taken away from us. I guess I was just really angry and bitter that others had the perfect life and ours had been shattered.

Keep a positive attitude. This is easier said than done, but vital to the role of a caregiver. There are going to be those days when your loved one is so sick she can't get out of bed. There might be times when her white blood count drops too low and infection sets in. Your loved one will probably lose her hair and gain a lot of weight. Depending on the treatment your doctor recommends, there could be an operation to remove a part of or the entire breast. You may find during the treatment that the cancer has spread to another part of her body. Depending on your financial situation, you may find that money is a very big factor in making decisions about treatment. There are many other things that will occur that will bring you down and keep you from that positive attitude.

During our time of fear, anger, bitterness, sorrow, depression and hatred of what we had been dealt, I never gave up hope. One look at my beautiful wife was all that I needed to keep me going strong and hoping for the best. Barbara's spirit and character gave me strength and courage. She faced the cancer with complete confidence that one day, it would all be over and we could get back to the happy routine that we both cherished so much. Granted, it would be a different life, because we would always live with the fear that the cancer would come back. But we vowed to each other that we would take it one step at a time. And the saddest part of it all was that we had very few choices except to do exactly what we were doing at the time. There was no magic cure.

All of this and more falls directly on the shoulders of the caregiver. Will it stress you out? Of course it will. But keep in mind that the crisis can be dealt with efficiently. Keeping the patient comfortable, informed and getting the best care you can provide are of paramount importance. Everything else takes second place. Keep in mind at all times that breast cancer, no matter what type, is a very dangerous and deadly disease. When you feel overwhelmed, reach inside of yourself for strength or call that friend whose job is to look out for you. If you practice a religious faith, relying on your beliefs can help.

Don't expect to be perfect. You will make mistakes along the way. But learn from your mistakes, and improve. Don't dwell on them too long. Make adjustments to your plan and move forward. It takes time to learn how to be a successful caregiver. Believe me, your loved one will appreciate every little thing you do for her.

And the simplest thing—but one of the most important—is to simply say, "I love you."

Thomas Brown is the author of *Men Bleed Too: A Compelling Story About One Man's Struggle to Help His Wife Fight Breast Cancer*, which chronicles his role as caregiver to his wife Barbara. His follow-up book, *She Taught Me to Laugh Again*, details life beyond the grieving.

Haunted By Dr. Love

Naomi Heilig

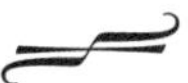

I lost my mother to breast cancer when she was forty and I was five. By my late twenties, I had become vigilant about prevention and started seeing a breast surgeon, Dr. S, twice a year. Three months before I turned fifty, he pronounced my latest mammogram "fine," then called me back in for a reexamination of an unclear area. Probably only scar tissue, he said, but he would get another opinion. On my next visit, the area had become "suspicious." I made an appointment for a biopsy.

Opening my eyes in the recovery area, I glimpsed Dr. S across the room. I heard him say to someone, "...a benign tumor that looked just like cancer."

My lump?

He walked to my bed and said, "Unfortunately, the machine is broken. We won't have your results for several days." My boyfriend, Michael, approached my bed and asked, "This hospital has just *one* machine?"

The doctor called three days later, urging me to come in as soon as possible. Michael and I rushed to his office. Dr. S greeted us, unsmiling.

"Well?" I asked. "What are my results?" Dr. S withdrew a sheet of paper from a manila envelope. Handing it to me, he said, "Here. Read them." I was a reading teacher, but the document's densely typed paragraphs overwhelmed me. He noticed this, and said, "Read the final diagnosis."

I couldn't find it. He took it back, did something with a magic marker, and gave it back to me. FINAL DIAGNOSIS popped out from within a black circle. I recognized the word *carcinoma*, the meaning of which I knew, lost among others with fuzzier meanings, like *intraductal*. He got up from his chair to refer to a wall chart of a breast in cross-section. I heard him say I had three choices: excising the lump, mastectomy, or bilateral mastectomy. He said I needed an immediate bone scan, liver scan, chest X-ray and blood work.

I reassured myself aloud, blurting, "I can handle this," while thinking, *I'm going to die and I'm not even fifty. I don't believe this!*

The doctor said he expected the four tests to be clear. Michael asked the prognosis.

"Good."

"Not excellent?" I asked.

"Prognoses are described only as either good or poor."

Oh.

"And the tumor's size?" Michael asked.

"Two point three centimeters, this puts her in Stage II."

"How could it grow like that in a year?" I asked. "You said my mammogram last year was fine." He offered to show me last year's film, but what was the use? I asked what he thought I should do.

He recommended a mastectomy.

I gasped, "Why not a lumpectomy?" "Your tumor is very deep inside the breast," he said. "It is difficult to reach. Doing a lumpectomy to reach it would be like coring a pineapple. You would lose your nipple, and enough of the breast, that I would not be able to give you an acceptable cosmetic result. And you would need six weeks of radiation. With a mastectomy, the breast would be reconstructed immediately. I would refer you to an excellent plastic surgeon who takes your insurance, and you would avoid radiation. But there's another reason I recommend mastectomy. If you chose lumpectomy, how would I follow you in the future? On an X-ray, cancer looks white, and radiation looks white. If you should have a recurrence of cancer after the breast was radiated, I could miss it."

He scoffed at Michael's suggestion that we get another opinion, saying it would just confuse us. When we insisted, the doctor scribbled a couple of referrals on a paper and thrust it at Michael.

Where to go on a Friday afternoon in spring, after a cancer diagnosis? We were near Union Square, which was abuzz with people having fun, talking on cell phones, making weekend plans. We ended up spending two hours cross-legged on the floor of the nearby Barnes & Noble bookstore, studying breast cancer books. Something I read that evening, in *Dr. Susan Love's Breast Book*, struck me. It was about being pressured to make a decision after a diagnosis about getting rid of your breast and thinking you can live without it, realizing only later that you really did want your breast.

The four tests turned out clear, meaning the cancer hadn't spread. After consulting Dr. S's plastic surgeon, I accepted that I would end up with two smaller breasts that would almost match, although only *some* of the reconstruction would be immediate. After surgery, I would awake with a makeshift breast, smaller than the one it would replace. It would be augmented in stages, through several surgeries, over months. At the end, it would not be as large as it had been. The healthy breast would also be reduced, so that both would match. Dr. S had not even hinted at this.

I convinced myself that afterwards, I'd look almost the same with clothes or without. This mattered to me. I was often told that my figure was beautiful. I loved shopping for clothes. But what choice did I have? I could do this, and I would do it, even though Dr. Love's paragraph haunted me. I cried when Michael held me and sighed, "My beautiful Naomi—you'll always be beautiful to me." He must have been imagining me bald, with one breast.

But my mother had gone through a mastectomy and so would I. Since my diagnosis, I'd thought of my life as a template laid over hers, matching it. My father felt the same way about her that Michael does about me. Michael loves me the same way, often purring sweetly about the smallness of my body. It's a copy of my mother's. (She once worked as an artist's model.) Another match, inspiring another man in love to feel protective as well as passionate.

With such support, how could I die? Michael and I became more "we" than ever. We repeated to each other that we would endure this together, as if this promise would guarantee my survival. But when Michael showered and could not hear, I sat at the dining room table, crying loudly into my crossed arms. My father's pain after my mother's death was my model of love in childhood. Now their story was my model of how Michael and I would endure this together. My empathy for my father's anguish remained vibrant, throughout several decades, available for my examination under the powerful magnification of an intensely felt crisis. When Michael said, "This is killing me," I thought of my father, whose eyes reddened and began to tear during the rare times he tried to talk about my mother.

I have been protesting that I was "all right" ever since my father told me of my mother's death when I was five. I'd replied then that he shouldn't worry, because we'd get another mother. At that moment, I became an expert at cheerfully, even inappropriately, insisting on the positive slant of tragic circumstances. I refused to abandon this automatic response now; it had always worked so well for me.

I felt detached from the upcoming surgery and I took it much too lightly, throwing all my energy into pretending I could handle it. I insisted that I no longer valued my breast, since it had turned cancerous. Still, I wore revealing tops every day, compelled to show off what I was about to lose. I convinced myself that after breast reconstruction I would still have the same body that others praised.

People remarked on my upbeat attitude, as I insisted on the positive side of cancer. Cancer allowed me to get away with anything. I reveled in the attention that it brought, the flowers that filled our one-bedroom apartment, the constantly ringing phone, the gifts, the little privileges I got by telling people I had cancer: I'd gotten out of a course assignment just by saying the word. Yet, I snuck glances at women's breasts, barely allowing myself to think: *they get to keep theirs; why can't I keep mine?*

Michael insisted that we meet two other doctors. One, Dr. D, the chief of breast surgery at an excellent hospital, said that a mastectomy was not called for and that a lumpectomy would not be disfiguring, as Dr. S had implied. He stressed that both procedures produced the same high survival rate after five years. We returned to Dr. S with more questions.

"The other doctor can be cavalier because he's not the one who's going to follow you afterwards," Dr. S began, not acknowledging that *he* had recommended Dr. D. "Your breasts are very dense, difficult to read on a mammogram. Remember, with lumpectomy, you need radiation. Cancer and radiation both appear white on a mammogram. I could miss a recurrence, unless I give you a mastectomy. At your age, forty, you have years ahead when cancer could recur."

How could he have missed that I was forty-*nine*? Still, I shuddered at his projection. We asked all our questions, heard all his answers, and again, I came away convinced that a mastectomy was the best thing.

The mastectomy was scheduled for a Monday at 8 A.M. with Dr. S. The Friday before we waited two hours for an appointment with Dr. B, chief of breast surgery at the world's most respected cancer hospital. We met him at 5 P.M., as others were starting their weekends. He labeled Dr. S's position "old-think." Dr. B assured us that other examination techniques besides mammography, such as MRIs, were available and that he could give me a cosmetically acceptable lumpectomy. Dr. Susan Love's words floated by, hovering over me.

"When?" I asked.

"I'll get my book," said Dr. B. Those words saved my breast.

Seven years after my lumpectomy, my formerly cancerous breast matches its mate, except for a puckered scar around the nipple. I go for checkups twice a year at the hospital where I had surgery. I never returned to Dr. S.

My mother kept a diary. She wrote that she would like to have written an advice book for women with breast cancer. She felt she had gotten very poor care. Although her cancer was diagnosed fairly early, her surgery had inexplicably been put off until it was too late. If only she could have known that, unlike her, I have survived the same disease with my breast and my life intact.

Naomi Heilig is a retired New York City public school special education teacher. The holder of graduate degrees in early childhood education and in French language and literature, she also trained as a professional cook. She attended the Vermont Studio Center on a writing grant and her work has appeared in *The Healing Muse*. A native New Yorker, she is currently completing a memoir.

Continued from page 186

Complementary and Alternative Medicine (CAM)

When someone is diagnosed with any kind of cancer, they want to do whatever they can to fight the disease. Some people will turn to complementary or alternative medicine. These therapies are considered to be outside of the standard treatments of chemotherapy, hormonal and immunologic therapy, surgery, and radiation therapy and are used in conjunction with these more generally accepted therapies. Some types of CAM include herbal medications, dietary supplements, acupuncture, massage, reflexology, reiki therapy, and tai chi, to name a few. A patient must be forthcoming with her doctors about her decision to incorporate CAM as part of her treatment. Many herbs and dietary supplements may counteract the effects of the standard therapies. Be aware that, although the term "herb" sounds milder than "chemotherapy," there is some overlap between the two: some chemotherapeutic agents are derived from plants that are popular with herbalists. Herbs are also unregulated and can be administered without the approval of the FDA. Some can cause serious side effects such as liver damage and bleeding, and because the herbs are readily available, patients will often self-medicate. With proper use, CAM can have many benefits, but it needs to be carefully incorporated into the treatment plan.

Continued on page 224

Part VI

I AM A SURVIVOR

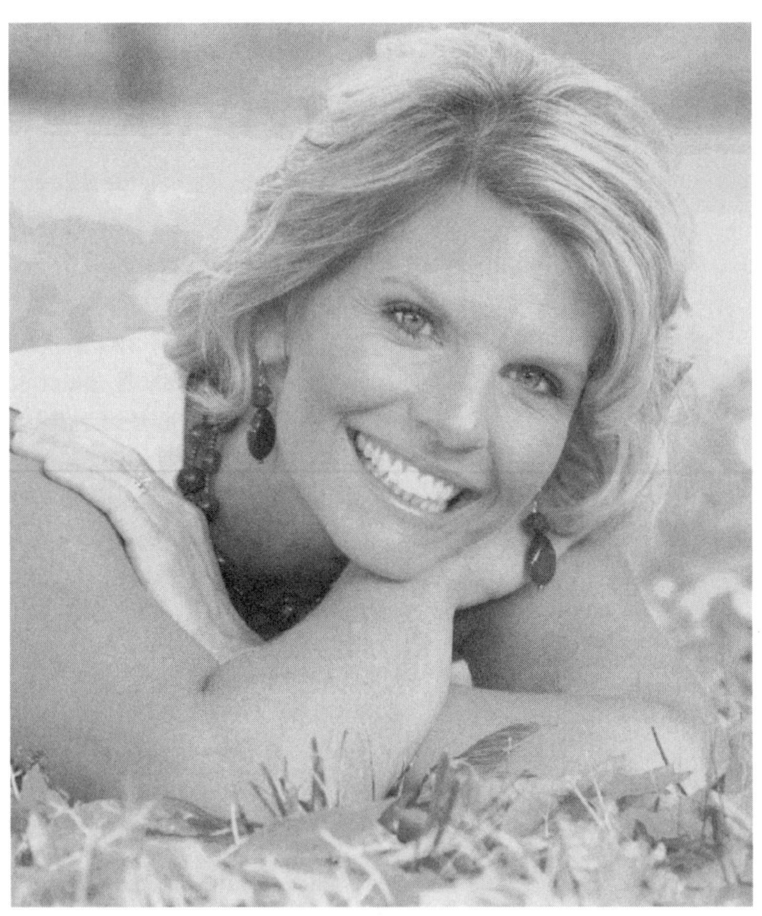

Tracie L. Metzger

The Pink Ribbon Girl

Tracie L. Metzger

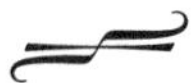

Certain phrases I've heard over the course of my life have greatly affected me:

Treat others the way you'd like to be treated. Knowledge is power. Will you marry me? It's a boy, it's a girl... But none has affected me so much as the one I heard on September 8, 2000: *You have cancer.*

Lying in the recovery room after what was supposed to have been a routine lumpectomy, I tried to focus on Dr. Columbus as she walked in, but I couldn't because my contact lenses had come out before surgery. She moved slowly across the room and didn't say a word. She sat down next to me and held my hand.

"I'm so sorry Tracie, but the lump was malignant."

At first I couldn't remember if the word malignant was good or bad, but I found myself sobbing uncontrollably once I figured it out. My husband Ray walked into the room and he knew it wasn't good news. He looked at Dr. Columbus and said "Cancer?" She nodded. I was in the middle of a nightmare but somehow I was able to pull myself together to ask, "Okay, what now?"

Dr. Columbus explained that she would go back into my breast to remove any remaining cancer tissue and then sample some lymph nodes to make sure it hadn't spread. Ray was a resident physician at the time and asked all of the pertinent medical questions: "Who do you recommend for an oncologist? Will she need chemotherapy? What is the survival rate?" All I wanted to ask was, Am I going to die? Will I lose my breasts? Will I lose my hair?

Then the faces of my two children, Trey, age 3 and Grace, 11 months, entered my mind. How would I tell them? Was I going to be able to take care of them during all this? I was their Mommy and no one else could do the things I did for them. Dr. Columbus assured us that I was going to be fine and told me that, although it was uncommon, I was not the only 30-year-old breast cancer patient she'd treated.

Calling my parents to give them the news was one of the most difficult things I've ever done. Not only because of the nature of what I had just learned, but because my younger sister had given birth to her first son the night before. I planned on heading up to the maternity ward right after my procedure. But instead I found myself on the phone, struggling to get the words out. "Mom, it's breast cancer." To hear myself say those words out loud made it all too real for me. I guess I was holding out hope that Dr. Columbus had made a mistake and confused my results with the poor girl in the room next door. "Don't cry Mom," I said, "I'm going to be fine. I'll beat this." And as difficult as it was to tell her that I had cancer, I found those words came easily for me. I believe that it was the grace of God working through me and I would handle this through faith, strength and a positive attitude.

My oncologist, Dr. Randy Drosick, saved my life. Of course, as a doctor he helped save my body with chemotherapy, but as a person he had an even greater impact in helping me handle the emotional side of this diagnosis. His wife had been diagnosed with breast cancer six months earlier and I believe that experience gave him a unique perspective in the way he treated me. Unlike other oncologists, he was able to say things like "I know how you feel," and I knew that he did. As a father of two children himself, he offered insight, support and encouragement to Ray. I think Ray looked up to Dr. Drosick and could relate to him on several different levels—physician, father, and husband of a woman with breast cancer.

Over the course of the next couple of months I endured chemotherapy, lost all of my hair, and had plenty of bad days. One time, I remember walking into Dr. Drosick's waiting room and felt like every pair of eyes was on me. Why wouldn't they be? I was at least twenty years younger than most of the patients in there. I asked Dr. Drosick if he had any other young patients I could talk to. The only women I knew with breast cancer were friends of my mom and they had been diagnosed in their fifties. Dealing with breast cancer while having kids still in diapers seemed a world apart from what these women were going through. I felt isolated and alone. I longed to talk to someone, anyone who could relate to the way I was feeling.

Not long after that, I caught a break. A friend of mine introduced me to Dawn Harvey, a woman close to my own age who had been diagnosed a month after me. Our first conversation was a bit awkward, mostly because we were complete strangers and were talking about breast cancer. But after a few phone calls, things went much smoother and I found reassurance and comfort in just hearing her voice. There was nothing like being able to talk to someone who knew exactly what I was going through. After several weeks we decided to meet.

I had started to look into the community for breast cancer support and found out there was going to be a meeting on Dawn's side of town. I asked her if she wanted to check it out with me and offered to pick her up. When she opened the front door I gave her a big hug. "It's so nice to finally meet you" I said. "You too," she said, "and I love your wig!" In the car we talked about anything and everything except our cancer, and we were both alright with that.

I realized that cancer was just one part of who I was, it didn't define me.

The next few months seemed to go by so slowly. It was the middle of winter, the sky was always gray, and the cumulative effect of the chemotherapy was wearing me down. I was clinging to thoughts of spring and the end of my treatments. By then, I would be finished with eight rounds of it and ready to undergo my surgery for a double mastectomy. Dawn and I continued to get together every couple of weeks and relied on one another for moral support. We talked about how lucky we were to have found each other and wondered what other young women were doing for help and support.

Springtime came and having the chemotherapy behind me was a huge milestone. I was ready to find a "new normal" for my life. With each passing day, I could literally feel my body coming back to me. I know that sounds odd, but imagine for a minute that your body is getting belted with chemotherapy, every three weeks for six months, killing almost every fast growing cell in your body. Then all of a sudden it stops. My tired body was thanking me with each passing healthy day.

The further we got from the end of our treatments, the more Dawn and I talked about other young survivors. Our oncologists had given our names to a few women who had recently been diagnosed. When I talked to them I tried to offer some encouragement and advice, but most of all I just listened. It was strange in a way, having someone look to me for the answers to the same questions that I had myself just six months earlier. But I knew that I was helping them and found myself growing through those relationships.

During the summer months of that same year, Dawn and I gave serious thought to reaching other young women and developing some sort of support network. We knew we had the drive and desire to make it happen. We chose October, National Breast Cancer Awareness Month, to send out letters to our local papers and television stations. Almost everyone agreed to cover our story.

I got a phone call from Dawn on the night before our first interview. I could hear the excitement in her voice when she told me about a crazy dream she had the night before. "I dreamed we called ourselves Pink Ribbon Girls." For weeks, we had been racking our brains trying to come up with a name for our group. We wanted it to sum up who we were. Pink Ribbon Girls—it was perfect.

We had the first official Pink Ribbon Girls meeting at Wild Oats Cafe and seven women came. It warmed my heart to see this group of bald young women sitting around a table, drinking coffee, sharing some laughs, some tears, and everything in between. It was one of the proudest moments of my life.

The monthly meetings have continued over the past five years and our numbers continue to grow. Today there are over 350 Pink Ribbon Girls and we are a nonprofit, 501(c)(3) organization. Pink Ribbon Girls are young breast cancer survivors who are encouraged by their shared experiences to educate and inspire others to grow and live beyond breast cancer.

I am proud to say that my "new normal" has changed again. Since my diagnosis I have had two more healthy children, Hope and Jack. I am a woman who wears a different hat on any given day—carpool mom, PTA member, soccer coach, President of Pink Ribbon Girls. Each role has its own merits, one no more important than any other. My journey down this road has been a true blessing in my life. The people I've met, the knowledge I've gained, and the lives I've touched have made it all worthwhile. Today there is one phrase that impacts me more than any other: *I AM A SURVIVOR*.

Tracie L. Metzger is the co-founder and President of Pink Ribbon Girls, a support network for young women diagnosed with breast cancer. She is active in the breast cancer community and was the first recipient of the "Patients of Courage Award" given by the American Society of Plastic Surgeons in 2003. She spends time speaking publicly about young women with breast cancer. She resides in Cincinnati, Ohio with her husband and four children.

Happy Birthday

Stephanie Davis

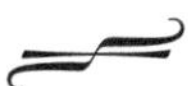

I was born in New York City in the mid-fifties; that's my legal birthday of record. However, an unexpected turn of events led me to create a different and more memorable version of my birth.

On the morning of October 23, 1998, as I sat at my desk, seven words changed my life. "You have malignant cells in your specimen," was the way Dr. Berlin informed me I had breast cancer. I heard nothing else he said after that, and my co-workers heard only my broken sobs as I rushed from my office to the hospital. There I was, at age 44, smack in the middle of a medical work-up to donate a kidney to my sister, and now I had to shift gears and face my own life-threatening (or life-saving) drama.

During a second biopsy—to prove what we both already knew—the doctor explained that I faced at least one operation (I had two tumors in the right breast), chemotherapy, and possibly more, if I chose to accept his recommendations. Well, accept them I did, and the experience was all I feared and then some. The overwhelming post-operative pain, unrelenting nausea and the loss of every, and I do mean every, hair on my body could not stop me from imagining the breast that had nursed my children lying fallow in a shiny aluminum pan. My nails had turned a scary shade of black, and it felt like an army of sores had invaded my mouth.

During that winter of recovery, I started in darkness and disorientation, and was pulled into the light of consciousness, sometimes kicking and screaming, sometimes praying, and sometimes smiling the silly, drugged smile of a newborn. I learned to sit up and walk with help, and learned to eat solid foods again. In my support group, I learned how to make new friends, take turns and appreciate diversity within a shared experience.

During "adolescence," I strengthened relationships long neglected and found love where it had always been. In my "adulthood," I went back to work, providing care to those who had cared for me. I guess I'm now a "senior citizen," providing information and assistance to those going through the process, the sage in the group who's seen and been through it all.

And that's why, on October 23, 1999, I found myself at the best one-year birthday party of all. Under a crystal blue sky, I sat tingling in the front seat of a small airboat, slicing through the Florida Everglades. I knew this was either the height of bravery or the depths of stupidity. I've had a lifelong fear of the water, can't swim a stroke and never even thought about going on thrill rides! However, on that day, far away from all that was feared and familiar, I was reborn. It didn't matter if I thought I saw an alligator or two. In fact, I didn't even flinch when the captain's wife shouted after us in her deepest Southern drawl, "Remember to bring 'em back this time, Bob!"

I was alive. Happy Birthday to me.

Stephanie Davis is a registered nurse living in New Jersey. Diagnosed at age 44 with Stage II breast cancer, she now lives "from a place of faith and gratitude." She has used her experience to reclaim her spiritual center and educate women about the value of early detection and intervention. Stephanie has been married for 27 years to Michael Davis, and has two children, Samantha and Christopher. She thanks her family and "sisterfriends" for their love and support.

Stephanie dedicates this story to the memory of her sister, Andrea, who unconditionally supported her, despite struggling with her own, terminal illness.

Taking Risks

Anthonine W. Carter

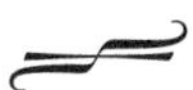

Breast cancer? Me? Why do I not feel surprised?

I think I know right from the start, when my annual screening mammogram shows a spot that is different from the study performed last year. My family physician orders another X-ray—this one called a diagnostic mammogram, for only the left breast.

I speak briefly with the radiologist who reviews the X-ray before I leave the clinic. He seems very noncommittal, almost evasive. "I can only say something is there that wasn't seen a year ago," he tells me. "At this point, I can't give you any idea about what this represents. Further studies will be necessary before I can say any more."

On the drive home I think about what this means and how it is going to affect my life. I think about how this winter has been subtly different from previous ones. For months I have wondered why my bed always felt so warm at night. For the first time in my recall, I have slid between the sheets on cold nights and found my feet were as warm as the rest of my body. Now I suspect that cancer has been growing in my breast, stimulating body metabolism which enhances the tumor's growth and results in a higher temperature.

The further study the radiologist referred to consists of a needle biopsy done with X-ray imaging. I feel apprehensive about the prospect of having a long needle inserted deep into an area as sensitive as my breast. Surprisingly the procedure is performed without pain and lasts only about forty-five minutes. Moderate bruising and tenderness are the only symptoms I experience in the aftermath.

Two days later I call the laboratory and learn that the preliminary results are completed. I can pick up a copy if I appear at the lab with a picture ID.

I make the short trip to the laboratory, but there is no doubt in my mind as to what the report will show. When the clerk checks my ID and hands me the paper, the pathologist comes forward and says, "You have ductal carcinoma in situ. Do you have any questions at this time?"

I tell him "No." Then without pause I say, "Thank you, thank you very much," as I turn to leave. Why do I thank him for telling me I have cancer?

When I get back in the car, I study the one-page report carefully. Right there in black and white the words stand out: "Ductal carcinoma in situ in all seven specimens submitted."

On the drive home I decide to stop for a visit with a friend. The first question she asks me is, "Have you been on hormone replacement therapy?" I control the urge to snap at her, to say something hurtful and sarcastic. Instead I remind her of the many times we have discussed this very thing; after my hysterectomy sixteen years ago, I began taking a low dose of estrogen every day, on the advice of my gynecologist.

Still she persists, and her voice betrays criticism and blame. "But why didn't you stop when all those researches were released to the public, showing that HRT is a contributing factor to the incidence of breast cancer?"

"I don't have complete confidence in all of those statistics and researches," I say. "Many of them are faulty, and sometimes they reverse their findings within a few years. I tried once to stop taking estrogen and found that I didn't feel nearly as well as I did during the time I was using it."

"I know—it kept you from aging in appearance, didn't it?" she observed. "Kept your skin from wrinkling and made you feel younger. My doctor wouldn't prescribe it for me. That's why I look so much older than you. And now I'm glad I was never on HRT."

For a brief moment I wonder what it is that keeps our friendship intact.

"No, it was the tired feeling I woke up with every morning without the estrogen. The swelling in my body, the peeling fingernails and dry hair ... the lack of energy all day. That's why I chose to take the risk. If it delayed the onset of wrinkles, I'm sure that was incidental. And yes, I've stopped taking it now." I remind her of the women we both know who have been diagnosed with breast cancer, several of them who never took estrogen, some who did.

I think about my friend when I arrive home. She drinks decaffeinated coffee because of her fears that the regular brand might cause breast disease. Then I recall the many risks I've taken throughout a long lifetime. I regret none of them. Living in fear simply isn't a lifestyle I've chosen. With each passing year, a woman's likelihood of cancer increases. Does that mean I should hope for a shorter lifespan to avoid that possibility?

I've made it a habit to take good care of my health—a physical exam every year, annual mammograms, regular visits at the dentist's and ophthalmologist's offices. And simply because I enjoy being active, I get plenty of exercise every day. There are so many wonderful people in my world—family, friends—and I look forward to every day that arrives. When I find myself alone, I have hobbies to keep me busy, and I enjoy a good bit of solitude because I like myself. I am confident with my life and my decisions.

My surgeon performs a lumpectomy and axillary node dissection two weeks later. The procedure leaves me with some discomfort and bruising for nearly two weeks. The drain is removed in five days, the sutures are out in ten days. The pathology report does not show any metastasis to the lymph nodes.

My doctor assures me. "This isn't going to get you, Tony. You've had surgery, and when your radiation and chemo are finished, you'll be well."

And I believe it, because I believe in myself.

I take risks.

I am not afraid.

Anthonine (Tony) Carter is a native of Maine, a retired nurse and septuagenarian. She now resides in the foothills of the Blue Ridge Mountains of South Carolina. She claims to be still growing up even as she grows older. She has had two books of verse printed for family and friends, *Reality Rhymes* and *The Barn And Other Poems*, a collection of short stories, *Lies And Half Truths*, published by Aventine Press, and she is presently putting the finishing touches to a debut novel as well as her memoirs.

Malignant Summer

Lauren LaRocca

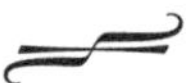

There were only two species of flowers for me that summer: the real flowers that were in bloom outside my window and the sad flowers in vases that filled my room, like a funeral.

I was cheating on my boyfriend that summer. It was the summer my parents split up, after my father found out my mother had been cheating on him with a guy at a trailer park near the river. My dad moped around the house and tried to pack up her things. I was 21, on painkillers from a lumpectomy.

A month before, a mammogram had detected a cluster of calcium deposits. There were cells, irregularly shaped and doing things they shouldn't. A biopsy revealed more specifics: I would need surgery. First my doctor told me alone and then my family and friends, like a doomed parade, marched slowly into the fluorescent-washed office to hear the news. My mother cried. My friend Abigail stared at the floor. I stared at my feet, which looked purple under the strange lighting.

They never say the word "cancer." Oncologists, surgeons, breast specialists, radiologists, they have a language of their own. Or maybe they think to disguise it helps their patients feel safe. Maybe they think if they put it in terms we don't understand, we'll feel like it's not real, like a dream, that we'll have nothing to connect it to. So they use their medical terms, neat and precise words I've never heard before. Words that mean nothing. They say *ductal carcinoma in situ*, in my case. But I wanted to understand, to connect with what I had.

So, I immersed myself in research—cancer treatment, cancer prevention. Pamphlets, magazines, books. I read them like they were survival guides. But they raised more questions than they answered.

Can you tell what stage they're in? If these harmful cells are within the ducts, could surgery break open these ducts and release them to spread? Is this why radiation is needed? Could radiation treatment give me cancer? Why can't we be born old and sick, and grow younger?

Invasive, non-invasive. These words are stronger: they tell you that a stranger with a sharp, foreign object will soon invade your body, cut through your flesh to see what's inside. The pain would come in quick, sharp spurts, and I would cry, hard and fast. Then I would be me again. "21/F" on my wristband, stitches in my nipples.

Nothing makes it feel real—not the fluorescent lights, not the statistics, not the anesthesia, not the pain pills that come following the surgery. Not the flowers that filled my bedroom, nor the cards or get-well wishes. My lover came over at two; we made plans to go to the ocean.

There is no written history of the cancer summer—the cheating, my best friend's abortion, my dad's depression which turned him to skin and bones, my brother's court dates before he was sent to prison. I destroyed all my notes—the only gap in my written history. Instead, my new lifestyle reminds me. I've gone from bags of chips to bags of rice, barley, and greens, from whiskey to green tea, from lazy afternoons to yoga practice.

It's three years later. I just got back from a sonogram appointment. The woman who did it was a breast specialist, so I told her my history, and she had an odd response.

"DCIS—that's like hitting the lottery!" she said.

At first, I thought she meant that the odds of me getting cancer at age 21 were so slim, so rare. But moments later, when I saw her beaming, I realized I was lucky, not cursed. I caught it, before it became invasive. I was lucky. I am lucky.

Lauren LaRocca is a native of Pittsburgh, Pennsylvania and works as an editorial assistant at *The Frederick News-Post* in Frederick, Maryland. She earned a Bachelor of Arts degree in Creative Writing from Warren Wilson College in Asheville, North Carolina and her work has been published in *Hagerstown Magazine* and *The Front*, among others.

Continued from page 203

Comprehensive Cancer Care

One of the greatest challenges for cancer patients, and especially the newly diagnosed patient, is managing all of their medical appointments. Dealing with appointments, treatments and tests located in different places around town is not only time consuming, but the added frustrations of scheduling, parking, traffic and potentially disjointed medical care increases the burden on the patient. It's a juggling act and it can be exhausting. In the 1980's, the idea of the comprehensive cancer center was born. In this environment, all services are delivered under one roof. A patient can have her surgery, chemotherapy, radiation, imaging studies and lab tests in one place. Most centers often offer nutritional advice, social services, support groups and, on occasion, access to complementary medicine. It can make a difficult time a little easier.

Do you have to seek care at a comprehensive cancer center? No, but if your doctors are under one roof, you can be sure that they talking to each other about your care so that everyone is on the same page. You want your care to be coordinated so that should problems arise, your doctors are informed and available to help.

Continued on page 254

Eva's Spirit

Leah M. Cano

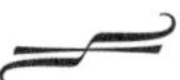

Our lives are made up of separate little stories. If we are fortunate, we learn how this seemingly unconnected string of vignettes fits together and we can see the plan, the purpose behind our lives. Someone whom I have never met helped me see how my life stories fit together. Her name was Eva.

I was a teacher in California, with literary aspirations and a deep desire to write and revel in a colorful Vermont fall, where the blowing leaves would inspire a multicolored flurry of words. But my aspirations were derailed when I got breast cancer. I felt like part of me had died. But another part of me was born. I like to think my cancer gave me new eyes with which to see the world and my part in it. I began to turn away from my frustrations and to appreciate my life more than I ever had. But a question, a doubt haunted me since learning of my disease and surviving it. I had never articulated it until, one day in my oncologist's office, I blurted it out:

"Why am I still here, when so many other breast cancer patients are gone?"

Once I had asked it, I was overcome with emotion. Why am *I* still here? Since I was given the opportunity to have this new life, there had to be some deeper mission to it: a new purpose that I was supposed to see, but couldn't. My oncologist answered, "Leah, that feeling will never go away, because you are a survivor. Many other survivors have this same feeling."

One weekend some time after my surgery, I arranged to go to a singles dance two hours away from my home. I planned to spend the night at a hotel with a friend. At the last minute she couldn't go. So I went alone. With no one to conspire with, I soon grew bored and left. Back at the hotel, lonely and a bit glum, I turned on the television. That's when I met Eva.

Eva Cassidy was a singer whose talent and life story had caught the media's attention. She possessed an angelic face and a voice to match. The report covered her rise in popularity, brought about by the indescribable emotion her singing could evoke. When I heard her voice, it seemed to me that her songs, her talent, came from a different world. Eva Cassidy was so remarkable; how could it be that she wasn't an international superstar? Apparently, she didn't want to be. When Hollywood agents came to see her, she wouldn't change her style to suit them. She insisted on remaining true to herself. And, despite her tremendous ability and devoted audience, she was so shy that she had to be coaxed onto the stage.

But something seemed amiss. The reporter only referred to Eva in the past tense. And then I heard it: Eva had died of cancer. I was overwhelmed by a rushing sense of connection with the late singer. She was one of those who had so haunted my mind—one of those who hadn't survived. The report ended with Eva singing a song that many said she had made her own: "Somewhere Over the Rainbow." Its lyrics of longing took on a new meaning for me.

I cried myself to sleep that night, thinking about Eva and her short life. She was only 36 when she died. In spite of my tears, I was glad that my friend hadn't come to the dance. Her absence had allowed me to discover this new friend.

Back home, I bought Eva's CD. I listened to it and was again moved to tears. I wished I had known her. There was something in her voice, perhaps the knowledge of her own looming mortality, that echoed the deep fears and yearnings my own cancer had left in me. I wished I could have shared my feelings of uncertainty with her. I knew she would have understood.

Some time later, listening to Eva's music as I ran on a treadmill at the gym, I decided to take a leave of absence from teaching so that I could regroup, refresh and write about my experience with cancer. As the song "Autumn Leaves" began, the words Eva sang took on new meaning for me. It felt as if she was singing directly to me. *The autumn leaves drift by my window. The autumn leaves of red and gold.* I had listened to this song many times since I first discovered her, but this time its meaning was different. It was as if Eva's spirit filled my heart with intense warmth. I saw in my mind's eye the leaves, their colors; I saw them drifting down on the wind. It was then that I fully realized how fortunate I was to have received this gift of a new life. I heard myself saying, "I must live each day of my life for those who could not." Here was my mission, the purpose that had eluded me since my surgery. My purpose would be to write, to try to encourage others and perhaps through my words give someone strength for their trials, as Eva did for me.

Perhaps it was just fate that soon thereafter I received a one-month writing residency in Vermont in September. Autumn leaves to help me remember and inspire me for the mission ahead.

Thank you, Eva.

Leah M. Cano is a teacher and writer living in Laguna Beach, California and has written for *Transitions Abroad* magazine, *MAMM*, and is featured on the *Experiment for International Living* and *Vermont Studio Center* websites. She finds it a mystery of life that her dream to become a published writer was realized primarily through her writings about her experience with breast cancer.

The Racer and the Singer

Phoenix Arrien

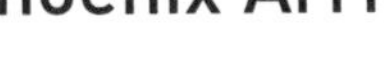

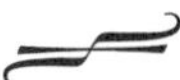

Michelle Hanton's chest heaves as the dragon boat plunges through the water, waves striking its sides. Arm and shoulder muscles bulge, strong fingers tightly grip the paddle, breaths come hard and fast, adrenaline surges and ears tune into the beat of the drum. The two rows of breast cancer survivors dip their oars into the water in unison as they plunge into the myth—that breast cancer stops you from using upper body strength—and watch it sink into the waves and out of existence. Michelle Hanton is a survivor. "I pound the water, feel the wind in my hair, feel a fire in my belly and my lungs burn," she says. "Then I know that I am still well and truly on this earth, that I am fit and I am alive."

Gia Pyrlis remembers crying uncontrollably. Having been diagnosed with breast cancer, she is having sessions with a psychologist between bouts of chemotherapy. In between the sobs, she hears the psychologist's calming voice say, "Gia, you are not going to die. You will be sitting in my seat one day helping other women with cancer." At the time she does not believe him. But now she realizes his prediction was correct. Gia Pyrlis is a survivor.

Michelle Hanton, dragon boat racer, and Gia Pyrlis, singer and counselor, are two Australian women who fought breast cancer and survived to inspire others.

Diagnosed with breast cancer in 1997 when she was 38, Michelle underwent a mastectomy followed by six months of chemotherapy. She found great inspiration from meeting other people who had survived cancer. "I accepted the challenges head on—along with moments of fear, self doubt and a lot of weeping—in the knowledge that others have also faced this. And if they could face it, then so could I. At the end of each difficulty, I would just pick myself up and think positive thoughts. Mindset is half the battle. I learned to focus on the present moment and enjoy it. I helped myself by meditating and drinking Kambucha tea. It might have been responsible for me not losing all my hair during chemo. I was also getting mouth ulcers from the chemotherapy and I met an old Chinese lady who suggested fresh paw paw, which I found worked well in healing the ulcers. I also looked after my diet and practiced meditation and visualization."

While going through her cancer journey, Michelle heard about the ancient Chinese sport of dragon boat racing from a Canadian who was involved in breast cancer survivor teams. With a crew of anywhere from 10 to 50, the dragon boat teams paddle in unison to the beat of an onboard drum, in racing competitions that are thought to date back 2500 years. She wanted to give it a try. So she rounded up a group of local survivors and entered a team in a local dragon boat competition. "I thoroughly enjoyed myself and wanted to keep going," she recalls. "There were no breast cancer survivor teams in Australia, so I joined a local mixed group. With the encouragement of the State Coach, I joined the State team heading to the National Titles in March 1999. The national competition became a turning point. It gave me a real thrill. I suddenly realized that I was starting to feel stronger and more in control."

Michelle found the experience so rewarding that she decided Australia should also have a survivor dragon boat team. She became the founder and National Coordinator of Dragons Abreast Australia. State teams were created and, by April 2000, they were able to field a combined team at the Australian National Titles with a crew who had never paddled as a team. "But we looked good in our hot pink lycra tops," she remembers, "and the crowds soon knew who we were and what our message was."

Since then, Michelle has left her pre-cancer career in manufacturing to work full time with Dragons Abreast. She has competed internationally and today there are dragon boat teams all across Australia. Wherever they go, they talk about breast cancer and encourage more breast cancer dragon boat teams. The racing helped Michelle become fitter and stronger, both physically and mentally. "When people are diagnosed with breast cancer," she says, "there are so many things you can't do: you can't lift and it's all very negative. Through dragon boating we have proved that we can do physical things including upper body actions. Racing dispels the myths and supports women in a positive way. Family and friends can also see us doing wonderful things. There are all sorts of women of all ages and all conditions in the same boat."

Michelle Hanson smiles with the serenity of a true survivor. "The essential element of dragon boat racing is the belief in the power to make a difference. Dragons Abreast is not about winning and losing races, it is about life and the belief that you can make a difference. We have fought the demon breast cancer. Many of us continue to fight, we do not lie down and accept this disease, we challenge it all the way. Every one of the pink ladies is a winner."

Gia Pyrlis was 33 when she was diagnosed with breast cancer. She had two children under the age of nine and her marriage of twelve years was failing. "Before I was diagnosed, I knew I wasn't happy. I had been a teacher for thirteen years; my marriage was ending and an inner voice was telling me that I was not living my truth. I was now facing the fear of death. I needed to make the commitment to begin my journey to live."

Gia looked deep into herself as the treatments began. A radical mastectomy of the left breast along with the removal of nineteen lymph nodes was followed by radiation therapy for five weeks, chemotherapy for five months and then the drug tamoxifen for five years.

"I was unable to face my body with its missing breast, so I decided to attend an eight-day retreat that changed my life forever. I began to identify my losses: the loss of my breast, the possible loss of my hair and ovaries (which didn't happen), the loss of my innocence, and the loss of what little self-esteem I had. Faced with a life-threatening illness, I was suddenly forced to face some truths. And I decided to commit to living."

One of Gia's first lessons was to let go of resistance and trust that everything was going to be okay. Gia always had a strong need to control things, but cancer encouraged her to let go of that need. "I needed to live fully, not a half life, and living my truth has emerged in acts of creativity and helping others." She took up singing in concerts and choirs, a lifelong passion that she had not previously pursued. "During the cancer process when I didn't feel well, I would get lost in the lyrics and my singing would really reach people and evoke deep emotions."

Part of Gia's surrender to trust was to let go of her marriage and to eventually divorce. Other friendships provided unconditional love and support. Gia found that talking to friends and qualified, empathetic people helped. "I needed to learn new ways and tools, so I had to learn to speak and think in a different language. This increased my positive thinking and meditation, visualization, exercise and leisure, especially leisure, all helped me let go." She also chose not to focus on cancer "percentages," because this type of information instilled fear. Instead she read, meditated and worked on changing herself from within. "One of the most significant things I learned to do is was to go within and listen to that inner voice. I still do it now when I get too busy. I go quiet, simplify my life and listen to that voice."

Gia's dedication to remaking the inner landscape paid off. She discovered a zest for helping others, and she has since earned a master's degree in counseling. She founded the first cancer support group for the Greek community in Australia. Gia has also opened a healing clinic where she practices remedial and therapeutic massage and counseling with the focus on cancer, preventative care, well-being and personal change.

Both Michelle and Gia are fully aware of the powerfully transformative effect breast cancer has had on their lives. Michelle says that above all else she has "learned to believe in myself and the power that each of us has as individuals to make a difference, and that collectively we are a force to be reckoned with." For Gia, her work now "encourages the mind-body connection and teaches me that we are our own best teachers."

Both women feel that one of the greatest blessings to arise from their cancer crises is their increased, enriching fellowship with others. "One of the most amazing moments in my life," smiles Gia, "occurred soon after my diagnosis. "My little boy looked at me in an amazed way and said, 'Mum, you've got new eyes.' Well, I have since gained many friendships...of people with new eyes." Michelle too has made wonderful friends. "It's a real tribute to the human spirit how dealing with something like breast cancer can bring out the best in people. A whole new world has opened up to me through dragon boating. I would never have found this without experiencing breast cancer."

Phoenix Arrien is a freelance writer and photographer who contributes health, travel, environmental and profile articles to publications around the world.

Just Three Months at a Time

Christina Dowling Olachia

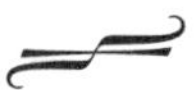

You have spent the last six to eight months as a cancer patient, just dealing with the day to day of cancer. Throwing up, nausea, no taste buds, exhaustion, pain in your bones, the list goes on. Now the chemotherapy treatments are over and you can say good-bye to the steroids. You are a cancer survivor. You take a deep breath and ask yourself, "Now what?" What do you do? Where do you go from here? Does it all go away and you just return to the once-sane life you thought you had? Well, not exactly.

Yes, you are now set free until your follow-up appointment in three months. That is a welcome relief. At least you have time to sort through the pieces of your life that have been scattered all over the place. Maybe you can get back to really cleaning and doing laundry? Maybe you can feel like cooking again or, better yet, eating again? Or maybe you will find yourself feeling more like a human being, rather than the monster that has taken over your body.

So three months it is! October comes, then November and finally December. Things look good. Yes, there are difficulties, but you have managed to get through a breast biopsy, a radical mastectomy, a port in and out, ER visits and six months of chemo, so you can definitely handle some minor issues. Then you start counting down the months again. If you can just get through to the next checkup, blood work and round of tests you will feel safe for another three months.

Your hair is coming back in; you actually have a face again with expression. Your swelling has finally started to go down (they left out the part about weight gain!). Your skin is on the mend and so are your taste buds. So you smile and depart the oncologist's office with a bit of hesitation: after all, you have been released to roam the world somewhat on your own now. So you muster up all your courage and take hold of this newfound confidence the doctor has given you and start your three-month countdown again.

Three months. Ninety-day intervals. It is just that simple. You are hopeful as you look to the future. You fully expect to watch your children grow from boys into men, to see them graduate, not just high school but college, and to see them marry and to hold your grandchildren pressed against your heart one day. But for now, you take life three months at a time.

The end of this month will mark my second three-month visit. From there, I will press onward and forward to my next three-month visit. For that is what they are, visits. Time to reflect on where I have been; embrace the staff that held my hand through each treatment, and time again to move forward to the next interval. So what will the next three months bring? Life and the living of life. Baseball season, basketball games, Easter with hair, an anniversary and another birthday. That is more than enough to be thankful for.

So I say, "Here's to three more months! Here's to living each of them one month at a time."

A longtime resident of Katy, Texas, Christina Dowling Olachia has been married to her husband, Johnny, since 1996 and together they have two sons, Joshua and Micah. With the support and encouragement of her family, friends and community, Christina has endeavored to live her life as a survivor filled with hope, laughter, strength and humor.

Celebration of Hope

Sheila Erwin

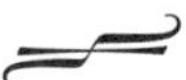

When I first heard that Kim, my sister-in-law, had been diagnosed with breast cancer, my mouth dropped open with disbelief. After all, she was a tough cookie who spent her forties experimenting with skydiving, white water rafting and other death-defying feats. Beating the odds with moxie had been the *modus operandi* for Kim, a popular reading teacher from Miami, until she encountered the greatest challenge of her life.

On March 21, 2006, freckled, red-haired Kim waited at her doctor's office for the X-ray technician to return with her mammogram results. The usual 30 minutes turned into an agonizing five hours, as more X-rays and sonograms were ordered. Then the doctor said the dreaded words. Something was unusual. He didn't know what it was, and he recommended a needle biopsy.

She was ultimately diagnosed with two malignancies. Her oncologist determined that it was Stage II cancer, located in two places, so a lumpectomy was out of the question. When she found out that she was going to need a mastectomy, Kim wept. Was she going to die? How would she tell her son?

"I did enough crying between April and June to last me a lifetime," Kim remembers. "Every day I would just break down, I was so scared of surgery. But I told myself that I was going to go through this without complaint and take it step by step. I kept telling myself that this was temporary and that I had full faith in my doctors."

Kim was in surgery for nine hours, cut from hip to hip and under her arms. A TRAM flap was performed: a surgical technique for breast reconstruction where the tissue, fat and muscle from the abdomen are relocated to the breast.

"I kept telling myself that I was going to heal," she recalls. "After my surgery, I was in the hospital for a week. Once I was able to sit up and move, I went right to the computer and started planning for the new school year."

When Kim returned to teaching she still looked the same, but once she started chemo her hair started coming out in clumps.

"When you start chemo, you lose your hair and the whole world finds out," Kim said. "I asked my son Vincent to shave the rest of it off. At first Vincent was reluctant, but I told him that I really needed him to do this for me because I couldn't do it myself. We went out in the back yard with the clippers and we both cried and laughed as he shaved my head to the skin."

After chemo, she returned to school with a bandana on her head. Eight teachers, two who are United Way coordinators, shaved their heads in support of Kim. Her students thought their teacher had shaved her head to be stylish until, during the morning address, the United Way coordinator announced to the 1,450 students that Kim had breast cancer. Kim broke down and cried when all the kids in the middle school dressed in pink in a show of support.

"I talked openly and honestly to the kids about breast cancer and about being a survivor," Kim says. "The kids see me as a human being, not just a teacher; they see that I have issues just like their families. The kids have given me hats, cards, books, hugs, opened doors for me and showed me great respect. They went home and told their families about me. The next thing I knew I was getting letters from parents saying, 'Bless you, I am praying for you, I am going through this too.'"

Kim, who had dreamed of being a teacher since she was seven years old, was recently elected Teacher of the Year for one of the regions of the Dade County School System. "Becoming Teacher of the Year has meant a lot to me," she says. "It has been a wonderful distraction and it's great to have the school recognize me."

Kim vows to continue the fight to raise awareness of breast cancer. Every October, Breast Cancer Awareness Month, she plans to call more attention to the disease and raise funds to help fight it.

"I know that I am going to be a survivor," Kim declares. "I am not on a five-year program. I am on a *50-year* program. I really believe I can beat this. When this is over, I'm going to have long hair again and tell my grandchildren about how I survived cancer."

Sheila Erwin is a mother, wife and freelance writer. With a Bachelor of Arts degree in Creative Writing from the University of South Florida, Sheila has been published in the *San Francisco Chronicle*, *Bloomsbury Review*, and *Autism Spectrum Quarterly*. Her mother, a 21-year survivor of breast cancer, taught Sheila how to be tough and face life's challenges straight on, but also taught her how to celebrate life. She does so by writing about others whom she admires.

The Lazy Days of Summer

Jacquie McTaggart

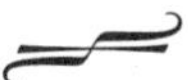

Everyone likes the lazy days of summer, when they can be outside and enjoy the treasures of the season, but teachers love them best of all. Teachers use their summer vacation to reflect, recharge and regenerate so that they can return to the classroom in the fall with the kind of vigor, vitality and enthusiasm that kids deserve. A teacher protects her days of summer fun and relaxation with a determination that silently says, "Don't intrude on my time. Don't send me to a meeting, don't ask me to chair a committee and don't demand that I get a physical exam. Let me return to the classroom to do what I love best."

Fortunately, that summer of 1989 the Independence, Iowa School District didn't care how much I grumbled or complained about using one of my precious early August days to get a once-every-three-years district-mandated physical exam. A rule was a rule and district administrators were not about to let me wiggle out of it.

Thinking about the golf match I was missing and mumbling nasty phrases under my breath, I angrily drove to our local family physician's office. What a waste of time this is going to be, I thought. Dr. Mochal will take my blood pressure, look down my throat and in my ears, do a breast exam, and tell me I'm good to go for another three years. I was wrong.

"Jacquie," Dr. Mochal said, "I feel a little something in that right breast. I really don't think it's anything to be too concerned about, but let's just check it out to make sure. I want you to have a mammogram." He wasn't smiling.

Suddenly, the thought of losing an hour from my precious summer day didn't seem so important. Wondering if I would be around to witness another summer, I made a little (make that BIG) deal with God. If He allowed me to see this thing through, I would never again gripe about the school district's physical exam policy. Shucks, I might even change my ways and have an annual checkup, if He'd just give me the chance. With tears streaming down my cheeks, I headed for the car and began what was to become a very long but lifesaving journey.

My breast cancer story is a bit bizarre, not because of its severity (or lack thereof), but because of some unusual twists and turns along the way. My first mammogram showed nothing abnormal or even questionable, but Dr. Mochal said he'd feel more comfortable if I got a second opinion. He referred me to a specialist in a nearby city. The specialist (after doing a manual breast exam) perused the mammogram I had brought with me and, like our local radiologist, saw nothing out of whack. "But," he said, "let's do a needle biopsy just to make sure we aren't missing something." That test was inconclusive.

He then recommended a surgical biopsy of the lump so that the tissue could be examined at the University of Iowa, but he said it was my call. The decision was a no-brainer: my stomach was in a constant state of flux, I was sleeping fitfully and in another week school would be starting. I had to put this issue to rest before I could even think about dealing with a classroom of wiggly, giggly first graders. We scheduled the biopsy for the following week, the day before school was to start.

The biopsy went off without a hitch and the doctor said his receptionist would contact me as soon as the results were in. I came home, worried, started school, and waited for the call. And I waited and I waited and I waited some more. Finally, ten sleepless nights later, I called the doctor's office and asked the receptionist what they had learned from my biopsy. Ten minutes and six Muzak songs later I heard her say, "I'm so sorry. Somehow the results of your test have gotten lost. I'll get on it right away and call you back as soon as I learn something."

Fifteen minutes later the phone rang, but it was not the receptionist calling. It was the Big Cheese himself. "Jacquie," the doctor said, "I want you in my office tomorrow morning, and I want you to bring your husband with you. You need a radical mastectomy, and you need it now. I'll transfer you to the receptionist and she'll give you a time." Click.

That was eighteen years and eighteen glorious summers ago, and as far as the doctors can tell, I might easily have eighteen more to go. I not only am cancer free, I am much wiser than I was the day I silently cursed my school district for requiring a physical exam every three years. God provided me with the strength and the courage that allowed me to get through that dark period, and I'm not about to renege on my part of the deal. I am much more diligent about doing my monthly breast self-exam, and I have an *annual* (no more of that every three years business) physical and mammogram.

Sometimes I'm asked if I find my annual checkups less worrisome now that I've been cancer free for such a long period of time. Unfortunately, I do not. On a day-to-day basis, I rarely think about my ordeal with cancer, and I certainly don't waste time waiting for the other shoe to drop, or more accurately—for the doctor to find cancer in the one remaining breast. But when checkup time rolls around, all of that changes. About a week before my scheduled exam, I get bitchy with a capital B. My husband used to ask me what was wrong when I would bite his head off for saying "Good morning" in the wrong tone of voice, but he no longer inquires. He has finally learned that I'm simply stewing about possibilities (rather than probabilities), and once I get the "all clear" report I'll be fit to live with again. For 360 days or so.

And what will happen if some year the report isn't what I want it to be? I'll meet it head on, confident in the knowledge that my abnormality was discovered early and buoyed by the fact that early detection saves lives.

Jacquie McTaggart lives in Independence, Iowa with her husband, Carroll. She has two sons, six grandchildren, and 1,500 former first grade students. Jacquie is an 18-year breast cancer survivor.

It Was Only a Breast

Teresa McQueen

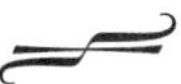

I would be forty in 2002. I was looking forward to this usually dreaded landmark. I had a dream job, a dream home a block from a lake, I was engaged, and my fiancé and I relished traveling in the beautiful Pacific Northwest region where I made my home. I was healthy and felt great.

But a painful lump in my right breast developed. My instincts screamed "cancer!" I frantically researched this possibility to prove myself wrong and, indeed, found that most resources noted fibroids as painful but cancerous lumps as not. With this information, I ignored my gut feeling and began monitoring the lump for changes with my periods or shrinkage when I quit drinking my daily pot of coffee. When my fortieth birthday rolled around and it was worse, I scheduled a mammogram. Five days after a stereotactic biopsy, I was told I had breast cancer.

I felt shocked disbelief and crushing aloneness with this diagnosis, despite it confirming my original instinct. I was certain it would prove to be an advanced stage of cancer. But I also somehow knew that it would not kill me. I unwaveringly decided on a mastectomy. After all, it was only a breast I was losing. My female family members, friends and acquaintances echoed this viewpoint. Many even said they would remove both breasts without hesitation. As expected, the pathology report indicated a Stage IIIb ductal carcinoma with thirteen positive lymph nodes. My oncologist informed me that even *with* treatment I had an eighty-percent chance of dying.

I still believed it would not kill me. It would be like my lifelong challenge with diabetes, from which I had no serious complications. Diabetes had only left me with built-up tissue due to my hypersensitivity to the insulin injections. So I was sure cancer would be the same. No death, just more deformities.

My emerging anger was not about a sacrificial breast. My new risk for lymphedema would exacerbate the restrictions on my inherently adventurous spirit already imposed on me by my diabetes. No more beloved nightly lobster-hot baths and getting my unprotected fingers buried in the dirt of my gardens. I was suffocated by the thought of this further onslaught to the quality of my life.

Wait a minute! I was going to survive cancer. How could these things weigh so heavily on me? I should be grateful to be alive, not angry. Despite my loved ones' support for me, guilt over my anger and fear kept me from sharing these feelings and I couldn't bear having even one person tell me how thankful I should be.

Instead, I devoured books and tapes about the cancer experiences of others. I was hungry for stories that would justify my seemingly ungrateful stance. The overriding messages were always about the cancer experience creating deep, spiritual self-change. This deepened my shame, for not feeling this. Then it hit me. I understood the nameless, nagging fear underlying my thoughts and feelings: I was deeply afraid that my diabetes-induced pragmatism would prevent me from experiencing any life-changing wisdom from my cancer. I felt incompetent.

I muted my fear in order to face my treatments. None of it was easy. I had an exceptionally long wait to remove the chest tubes from my mastectomy. I went to work unable to wear a prosthesis for months. I endured agonizing ice baths on my feet during one chemo regimen to avoid disabling blisters. I was nauseous, vomited, had diarrhea, constipation, joint pain, sleeplessness and hot flashes. I was exhausted to the point of feeling like I could not breathe, let alone lift myself out of bed to go to work or help around the house. I persevered in working through four and a half of my six months of chemo. I coped with the toxic infusions by envisioning that I had, amassed in every pore and every vein, cancer-killing Rottweilers bristling with bulging muscles under their shiny black hair. Their bright red collars represented the drugs.

When I lost my hair, I sported my bald head wherever I went. Women complimented me on my bravery to do so. But I was not brave. Whenever I considered wearing a wig or one of the beautiful turbans my sisters made for me, I became nauseous. They were an undeniable statement of my illness. I needed the public face of being a healthy, bald woman by choice. It was my desperate attempt at a reprieve from the daily reminders of my plight. But my demeanor clearly did not match my facade. Strangers flocked to me with their condolences for my cancer. I always went out believing I looked healthy and always found myself crushed under the reality that these well-meaning strangers would not let me forget.

As if the cancer and its treatment weren't enough, things got even worse. I discovered that my husband was having an affair. Marriage counseling started and I spent my radiation treatments all alone. No loving spouse by my side. The guitar serenade with roses he arranged for my last chemo was forever marred by the knowledge that those were days he was also lavishing attention on another woman. I was in an emotionally abusive relationship. Wow. Now what? I chose to take care of me and focus on my treatments. I took refuge over four hundred miles away in my parents' home. I'm amazed I managed to keep fighting as my imagined dream life disintegrated around me. My family's support proved invaluable.

After my year of treatments, I had a hysterectomy to rid my body of cancer-feeding estrogen. I moved out of state with the intention of getting back to work and to my life. I had a new relationship and bought a home. Unexpectedly, I started having increased joint pain, fatigue and "chemobrain." I learned my symptoms had a name: *cancer treatment late effects*. They disabled me from caring for myself, let alone my home or others.

Despite these challenges, I am honestly grateful. On most days, I am able to say that this journey was my wakeup call, to fully engage my attention to my life, my self. I had made so many choices that did not support my spirit and believed lies about who I was due to my own inner confusion. I was the perpetrator of my own victimization in so many ways and in so many relationships.

I began to write as I had when I was younger. It freed me to more honestly explore the fullness of all my emotions with my cancer and my life. It gave me the vocabulary, the introspective voice, for my reflections. I could finally express my despair in having lost so much. I realized cancer had allowed me to keep sight of myself. I allowed myself to mourn the loss of not just a breast, but my beautiful breast. The normalcy it had given to my shape, sexuality, and physical balance. Honoring its sacredness gave me a more peaceful path forward. With each additional word put to page, my spirit lifted and my soul, my self, was nurtured. My childhood dream of becoming a writer re-bloomed. At forty-two, though, instead of just dreaming about it, I actually began to do it! And so, yes, another cancer story is one with a reverberating message of enduring, life-changing awareness. The loss of my precious breast brought me back to my own truths of self-worth and life purpose. In my fourth year of survival, I am finally a believer.

Teresa McQueen is a registered dietitian. After a decade of interesting and successful career opportunities, her experience with breast cancer left her questioning the many choices made in her life. Her efforts to keep a journal of her experience contributed to her spiritual healing and rekindled her childhood dream of becoming a writer. She hopes her story can inspire others facing challenges in their lives. Teresa continues her cancer recovery and lives with her loving parents in Idaho.

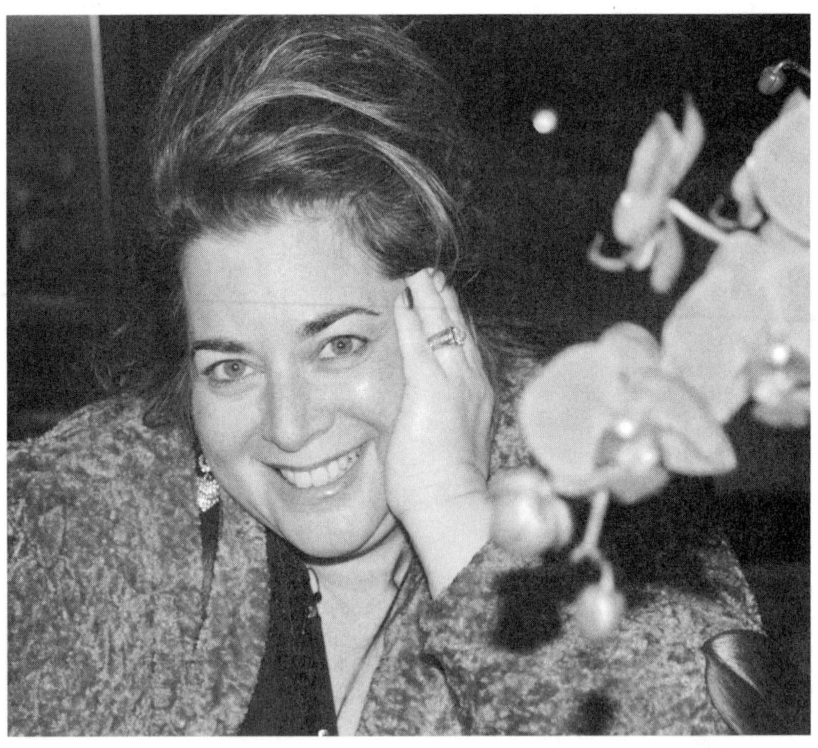

Laura Fial

Soul Survivors

Laura Fial

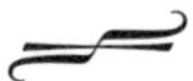

"Happy birthday, Laura. You have breast cancer."

Not the exact words from my doctor, but the timing of the diagnosis couldn't have been worse. And what a birthday it was: I was also dealing with my husband leaving me, being kicked out of my 10-piece music band, and my young daughter being diagnosed with a severe panic and anxiety disorder.

The oncologist, Dr. Quiet, gave me the news: "You have the good kind of cancer," she said. *Good kind?* Quite honestly, I didn't know there was a good or a bad kind. I thought cancer was cancer: horrible. How could losing a breast be good? I was crushed.

Dr. Quiet knew I was a professional jazz singer, always in the public eye, and that I ran a group that put together musical fundraisers for charities. Dedicated to helping the victims of this disease, Dr. Quiet was starting a nonprofit to benefit the cancer cause. She asked me to go home before starting my treatments and think of something I could do that gave me pleasure, passion, courage. I tried to calm down and listen as she told me to think outside myself, maybe think about something that would do some good for others who were going through this.

But, I reminded her, the fundraisers I helped with were for causes that were not about me personally. Everyone else had cancer, not me! Then she gave me the best advice anyone could get: "Please go home and come back with a positive attitude," she said, "I have sixty or so patients right now worse off than you but who are off the charts with positive energy." Wow.

I was ashamed. So I thought, okay, I am going to lose a breast. But I need to get through this. I *want* to get through this. I've been in music for over twenty years. Why not surround myself with positive women, women who are going through this same crisis? And sing about it! I would call my group the Soul Survivors—women who sing from their souls; women who sing about surviving. So that was it. I had a mission that would become my focus as I went through the frightening process of dealing with breast cancer. And the proceeds from the Soul Survivors would be donated to Dr. Quiet's foundation.

I decided to run a contest to find a song that would represent the concept of the Soul Survivors. I called a Phoenix newspaper, the *Arizona Republic*, to tell them about it. After my first week of treatments, exhausted, yawning, but crying tears of happiness I was interviewed by a reporter. The story ran on the *Republic*'s front page; by noon that day I had 70 calls from women all over the valley and a song for the group.

With the perfect song in hand and a roomful of musicians and singers, I held the first practice in my home with a person from the local NBC affiliate present and a Phoenix choir director to manage this massive group. To save money, we recorded our first CD in a friend's garage. We were thrilled to have a CD release party with an audience of 1,200 complete with food vendors, wine distributors and a silent auction. It was a magical night. I was exhausted but had met lots of new friends and the Soul Survivors were on their way to touching many people. Since then we've recorded more CD's, gotten lots of attention for the cause and yes, we've had a great deal of fun on our mission to heal through music. And focusing on the music and the mission of the Soul Survivors helped me through my journey as it has others in the group and as we hope it will help many others whose lives are touched by this disease.

I am now in the company of some tremendous soul survivors. I am getting married again, to a wonderful man, my singing career is very busy, my daughter is going off to college in the fall and doing very well, and I am cancer free. I may have lost a breast but I consider it a small price to pay for all I have gained.

Laura Fial is a professional jazz singer who lives in Arizona. She is the creator of the *Sing For Life Foundation*, the mission of which is to heal through music.

Continued from page 224

Taking Charge

Women with breast cancer face many challenges. Whether a woman is young or old, this is a frightening disease. The patient must take advantage of the many resources that are available for help along the way. As hard as it may be, keeping a positive, yet realistic attitude can make all the difference. There are advances being made every day that lead to more hope. As strange as it may seem, one should use the disease to take charge and to focus on the things that really matter in life. It is often through hardship that we see clearly and learn more about ourselves and of what we are capable. Breast cancer survival rates are good and are only getting better. Not everyone will survive breast cancer, but eluding death is not the benchmark of the victor, as everyone in this world will pass in time. The spirit of those who endure the disease with dignity and strength, and truly make the most of their time on earth, is the lasting mark of the winner.

Stephanie F. Bernik, MD, FACS, is Chief of Breast Surgery for the comprehensive breast program at St. Vincent's Comprehensive Cancer Center in New York City. A board certified surgeon specializing in breast diseases, Dr. Bernik further specializes in treating women under 40 diagnosed with the disease.

A 1993 graduate of Yale University School of Medicine, she completed her internship and residency at St. Vincent's Hospital and Medical Center in New York City. She was awarded fellowships at Memorial Sloan-Kettering Cancer Center in breast surgery and St. Vincent's Hospital and Medical Center in surgical oncology. Dr. Bernik also received two research fellowships from Yale University School of Medicine in 1990 and 1992. She received her undergraduate degree *magna cum laude* from Columbia University in 1989.

In 2005 and 2006 she was honored with the Top Doctor Award by the research firm Castle Connelly. In 2004, she received Columbia University's John Jay Award for Professional Achievement and in 2001, Columbia University's Alumna Achievement Award. Dr. Bernik is the author of many medical journal articles published in, among others, *The Journal of the American College of Surgeons*, *The Breast Journal*, *Journal of Nuclear Medicine*, *Annals of Surgical Oncology*, and *The American Surgeon*. She is a principal investigator for breast disease research at St. Vincent's Hospital and has presented her research at symposia across the country, most recently at the American Society of Breast Surgeons 2007 annual meeting and the American Society of Breast Disease 2007 annual symposium.

Sue Hunter's Story

Graham Mole

If ever anybody got to know the slough of despond, it was Sue Hunter. She'd just been divorced after seventeen years of marriage and faced bringing up two children as a single mum. Things were hard enough for her when, at 39, she developed breast cancer and had to suffer the ordeal of a mastectomy.

Sue recalls, "It was like being hit with a sledgehammer. In a split second the certainty you've always taken for granted has gone forever and your life is spiralling out of control. During the first couple of weeks I would wake up already crying; there was no getting away from the devastation, even while asleep."

She got through those weeks. The weeks turned into months, then years. But six years later Sue learned she had not left breast cancer behind. She was told there were problem cells in her other breast and quickly had an operation to get rid of them.

Afraid that there was no escape from the disease, Sue grew very depressed.

Then a friend of hers, Jim, invited her to go fishing with him, claiming that it would help her to get away from her negative thoughts. "I thought he was crazy," Sue says. "Why would he think I'd want to go fishing? I didn't want to be mucking about with maggots and worms! But he promised to buy me lunch and a couple of drinks so I thought 'why not?'"

Jim was right. "Within the day, it wasn't just the fish who were hooked: I was, too. Whenever I spent a day on the water I would come back in a very relaxed frame of mind—definitely a big plus when you've just been diagnosed with something like breast cancer."

Six months later Sue had to have a second mastectomy because the initial operation had been unsuccessful. She asked for the operation to take place as soon as possible because she didn't want to be out of action when the May fly hatches came due, a favourite time for anglers to be on the water.

After she had the operation, the first thing she asked her physiotherapist was, "When can I start fly fishing again?" Fortunately for Sue, the physiotherapist's girlfriend was also a keen fly fisher, so he had a good idea of what was involved in pursuing the sport. He told her that so long as she was protective of the actual wound site she could pretty much start straight away.

Sue is convinced that fly fishing aided her physical recovery as well as her emotional healing: "The action of casting helped me to regain movement in my arm. With the first operation, although the surgery was more drastic, I couldn't lift my arm properly for ages. But with the second operation I was out on the water within three weeks."

And the benefits went beyond the physical. "Fishing definitely helped with my emotional recovery in my second bout with breast cancer. It gave me a new focus, a positive challenge. Fly fishing gave me back a sense of control. Little things like deciding what fly I was going to fish, what line I would fish, where I was going to make the cast... I even learned about entomology. All these things had to be thought about, and in doing so I gave myself a very welcome break from thinking about cancer."

Sue also experienced a new and valuable relationship with nature, finding it very therapeutic to be near the water and to be exposed to the seasons. After her diagnosis, she found that she was noticing things in nature—like how green is the grass and how blue is the sky—things she had previously overlooked. Like most anglers, Sue found that just being by the water truly lifted her spirits. And even though fishing is a quiet and peaceful pastime, it gave her courage for her fight. She explains, "Out there, you're being bombarded with subtle information: it might be the weather or the water conditions, which insects are hatching, the season. You have to process all that information to try and beat Nature at her own game."

Sue Hunter has certainly done that. As she progressed in her recovery and in her new sport, she found herself transformed from a self-confessed "matching bag and glove girl" to a "tackle tart," more interested in the latest fishing gizmo than in the latest fashion. And her dedication to fly fishing paid off with the top-notch skills of a true sportswoman. Just a year after taking up the pastime, Sue made the England ladies' fly fishing team.

Now the former "matching bag and glove girl" has represented her country five times. She has seen England take gold medals in four of the five matches she has fished, and on each of these occasions she was also well placed individually. Finally, she was elected captain of the team, quite an achievement for someone who only began fly fishing relatively recently. But such are Sue Hunter's passion and dedication.

Sue has harnessed that passion, and her survivor's zest for life, to help other women who have been touched by breast cancer. The England Ladies' Fly Fishing Association—of which she's secretary—has been chosen to partner with the U.S. Casting for Recovery organization to extend the program to the U.K. and Ireland, running free weekend fly fishing retreats. Casting For Recovery allows women affected by the disease to gather in a beautiful, natural setting, learn fly fishing, meet new friends and have fun. Its retreats offer counseling and educational services to promote mental and physical healing. Casting For Recovery now has the backing of the Countryside Alliance and the U.S. tackle firm, Orvis.

So what is in fly fishing for women? Sue explains, "Women are very good at putting everyone else first, but this gives us time for ourselves. It's a real escape; you can use the time to think about the meaning of life. For women with cancer it is a real emotional therapy. The pleasure of connecting with nature can be so restorative."

And even though fishing can represent quiet times to get away from the world and reconnect with one's self and nature, Sue enthuses about the many social connections that it can inspire—connections that can speed healing and recovery. "Weekends are precious times," she says, "and couples and families like the chance to get out and do things together. Fly fishing fits the bill perfectly. It's such a social sport, you're virtually guaranteed to meet new friends. I met my partner David through fishing. What more could I have wanted?"

An award-winning investigative journalist and former TV producer based in the United Kingdom, Graham Mole writes on ecological and conservation issues for national daily and Sunday broadsheet newspapers and magazines. He has recently written an environment-themed novel and screenplay which have excited the interest of celebrities from the worlds of entertainment and politics.

Breaking Barriers

Beth L. Gainer

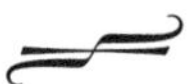

I didn't grasp life until I nearly lost it.

Six years ago, I was diagnosed with breast cancer. I was stunned. In addition to being only in my thirties, I was in overall excellent health and led a healthy lifestyle. Besides, my most recent routine mammogram was negative and my gynecologist had given me a clean bill of health during a recent annual checkup.

Looking in the mirror during my routine monthly self-exam, I noticed a very subtle dimple in my right breast. Over the next two weeks, I stared at the area in disbelief, hoping the dimple would just disappear. When it didn't, I insisted that my gynecologist re-examine my breast. He reassured me, saying that everything felt normal. But just to be on the safe side, he sent me for a mammogram at my hospital's breast center. During the procedure, the technician hurried in and out of the white, cold room, taking endless pictures of my right breast from every angle possible. By the time the radiologist came to see me, I already knew.

He said there had been a change since my last mammogram. But he tried to be positive, saying the abnormal mass found in my breast might not be malignant and that a biopsy was needed. After my biopsy, another doctor tried to allay my fears, citing statistics that, in premenopausal women, only one breast lump in 12 was malignant. The odds were in my favor.

On a bitterly cold January morning, I got *the* call. Breast cancer. Like many younger women, my breast tissue was dense. That's why my 1.7-centimeter tumor was missed by the routine mammogram. The doctors estimated it had been growing for eight years. To maximize my chance of survival and because I was young and fit, I received a brutal regimen of radiation and chemotherapy treatments simultaneously. Being proactive had helped save my life. Ironically, so did the cancer, but in a different way.

You see, by the time of my diagnosis, my personal life was spinning out of control. My husband had long stopped working, drained our finances, and isolated me from others. I was miserable at work as well, where I endured abuse from my overbearing boss and piles of overtime. Yet, rather than set boundaries on their behavior towards me, I passively accepted my plight. I became a recluse with little self-esteem.

Then came breast cancer and the brutal fight between life and premature death. Yet somehow, beneath the debris of suffering, I found an inner light, a voice—one of strength, courage and self-respect—that changed the trajectory of my life

Dead ends were replaced by lifelines as I sought to come to terms with the diagnosis and to deal with treatments. I joined several support groups and the American Cancer Society's Reach to Recovery program. For the first time in my life, this former recluse enjoyed talking to strangers. I was soon building a strong foundation of current and new friends.

I found unexpected heroes in unlikely places, such as encouraging co-workers, kind strangers at the hospital, the doctor who hugged me and held my hand, the nurse who gently wiped away my tears as she rocked me like a baby. And there were the superheroes—my parents, brother, aunt, cousin and friends who rallied around me and gave me strength, hope and courage. The phone calls that kept rolling in reminded me of how much I was loved.

And I needed their love and support desperately; I was terribly ill from the treatments. With my husband still refusing to work, I held onto my job and picked up another because of the ever-dwindling money supply, taking only one sickday throughout my treatments. I had no time to think. I was reduced to basic animal instincts: I needed to stay alive—despite a malfunctioning immune system, a faulty digestive system and immense fatigue and cognitive impairment. And to make matters worse, chemo-induced menopause destroyed my dream of bearing children. But my single-worst moment in an infinite sea of worst moments was a few days after one of my chemo treatments. I was rushed to the emergency room with a dwindling white blood cell count and a raging infection. The toxins had taken over my body and persuaded it to betray me. The hospital staff wheeled me into an isolation room, administered IV antibiotics, and barked out orders to wear masks around this patient with a suppressed immune system. This wasn't *ER*, and there was no George Clooney. This was *my* life. The doctors and nurses were so desperately trying to help *me*. I remember thinking, "So *this* is what it's really like to be ill."

Within a year after my last chemotherapy treatment, I rid myself of the remaining toxins—my husband, my unhealthy career and people who had rejected me upon hearing of my diagnosis. I felt lucky: I got a second chance at life and I realized that I hadn't fought so hard to live in order to be miserable. Breast cancer taught me a powerful lesson: I would no longer just exist; I would start to live.

Today, I live a full, content life. Like everyone else, I have bad days, but I view them as good days in disguise. I am happily divorced, financially independent and enjoying new hobbies and many new, true friends. I am about to embark on another significant journey: I am adopting a baby girl from China and finally realizing my dream of motherhood after all! I changed careers as well: now I love teaching at a local college, helping others. My work has been recognized by my colleagues and the community and I even won a national teaching award!

My greatest achievement, though, has been in my relationships with those I love. My family and I are closer than ever and we try to spend as much time as possible with each other. I surround myself with positive, kind, good people. I have a full social life filled with family, friendship and love.

But the relationship that has grown most of all has been that with me. I now advocate for myself, set boundaries on other people's behavior towards m, and I insist on being treated with respect by others. The cancer experience has changed and enriched my life in a way that I believe would otherwise never have occurred. Which leads me to the question that others often ask me: Do I view breast cancer as a gift?

I don't have an answer.

I would never have chosen this path. I still have days when aches and pains scare me. And while my doctors are all wonderful, kind and brilliant, I see them more often than I care to. There are days when I throw myself a pity party or two since I'm still dealing with breast cancer–related issues: as I write this, I am recovering from a preventive double mastectomy with reconstruction. Yet despite all this, I wouldn't trade my life for anything. It's been richer than I could ever have hoped for. I know individuals who, even after breast cancer, continue to impose barriers on their own happiness. To me, these survivors exist, but choose not to live. I decided to break the barriers to my happiness.

Originally from the Bronx, New York, Beth L. Gainer teaches college English in the Chicago area. She holds a Master of Arts degree from DePaul University and is at work on a book of poetry on the breast cancer experience from a younger woman's perspective.

LiveLoveLaugh

Donna Spillane

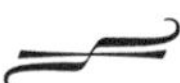

When you are dealt lemons, make lemonade. I know it's a terrible cliché. But every once in a while, the cliché fits. In my case, the sour situation is breast cancer. My story is how I, diagnosed with breast cancer four times over the past 15 years, have turned lemons into an ocean of lemonade.

In 1990 at the age of 30, I was diagnosed with breast cancer. It was a different time then; breast cancer was still not openly spoken about, treatments we take for granted today were still somewhat experimental, and public awareness of breast cancer was reserved for post-menopausal women.

My doctors performed a modified radical mastectomy and I was served up six months of chemo cocktails. I lost my glow but not my identity and after a short while bounced back to a relatively busy life, vowing to reconstruct my breast by my 40th birthday. I have always been goal-oriented, so I knew I would make my vow become a reality.

Over the next ten years, I climbed the corporate ladder and with each mammogram and blood test that came back negative, my breast cancer experience receded further and further away, a life-altering moment in time that had found its proper place in my memory.

I forged ahead with the belief that the cancer was behind me. My husband Kevin and I, with the help of fertility specialists and with the odds against us, gave birth to a beautiful baby boy. Life was good...a little unexpected, but back on track.

Happy birthday to me!!! Right on schedule, a few weeks before my 40th birthday, I began the reconstruction process on my right breast. A supermodel's bosom, that's what I wanted. A personal gift to myself. A badge of courage I would wear proudly! The reconstruction process went well, and I soon went on vacation. Little did I know that while I sunbathed, bikini-clad on the beaches of Aruba, my plastic surgeon was running pathology reports on suspicious cells he had uncovered during the reconstruction surgeries. I came back from vacation to find that the cancer had recurred in the chest wall of my right side—breast cancer #2.

My plastic surgeon saved my life. The reconstruction was reversed, the cells were removed and I went through seven weeks of radiation treatment. I was given a five-year prescription for tamoxifen and the countdown to survival began again.

I continued on with my life, engulfed in the chaos of motherhood and career, convinced that this was it; I had been dealt my hand, played it and managed to stay in the game. After all, how much should one person have to go through?

I've always been efficient and conscientious about my doctor visits, mammograms and blood tests. In fact, I've regarded them as somewhat routine. So, imagine my shock and devastation when I learned—from a routine mammogram—that now I had cancer in my other breast. Completely unrelated, the doctors consoled.

Mastectomy #3. Off tamoxifen. No additional treatments required. I convinced myself to think as if this was a first-time cancer, found early, completely curable. I healed and got back on track.

But not for long. Shortly afterwards, when I began the reconstruction process again, my surgeon discovered cancer cells, again on the right chest wall—breast cancer #4. The cancer was contained but the procedure to remove it was serious.

I would be lying if I told you I bounced right back from this news. I have extremely strong denial skills and I have decided to live my life, but this last diagnosis frightened me. I still went through the motions of a career and I embraced motherhood as my savior, but for the first time in a long time, I felt angry, defeated, and uncertain how I would handle this newest challenge.

Family and friends are the great healers and I got through the operation like a trouper. I have a wonderful rapport with my doctors and unfortunately, or fortunately, they treat me like an old friend. It's now over two years since my last cancer diagnosis. I fully recovered from all surgeries and, strange as it may seem, I am feeling motivated, strong, enlightened. And I am proud, proud to tell my story, proud that with early detection I am a survivor. Proud to know that with medical advances there will be more success stories like my own.

So I take each day as a whole, not looking back but planning ahead. Vacations. Family celebrations. Career advancement. I'll be there, every day, smiling and sipping lemonade from a pink straw.

A graduate of the Fashion Institute of Technology with a degree in marketing, Donna Spillane is the head of product development, production and sourcing for a leading men's and women's apparel company. Married for 21 years, she lives with her husband and son on Long Island's North Shore.

The Sky Is Falling!

Marie Fowler

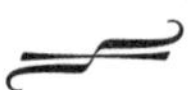

As if orchestrated,
The Muzak plays "One Moment in Time"—
And a life is forever changed.
The mammogram technician whispers,
"Good luck."

The physician, a healer,
Is uncomfortably cast as the bearer of dread
To a woman he has never met.
They are afraid of me.
Doubtless fearing a woman's hysteria,
He reschedules my appointment after office hours,
When no others are about.
Twisting in discomfort, the physician sputters out his curse,
Mumbling something about options.
Lost in the sea of terror enveloping me,
"The bottom line is," I manage to croak,
"My little boy is only seven."
The sky is falling!
Cruel surgery comes and goes, slicing into my private self.
The body that was mine alone—
Now paraded and pummeled by a thousand staring hands,

Cold and knowing.

The oncologist arrives, clipboard in hand.
He stops to smell the flowers, making me unaccountably angry.
You have the time and I don't.
"Someone cares a lot about you," he begins,
Fingering a velvet peony, staring out the window,
Unable to face me.
"It's my birthday," he finally mumbles, "I'm *40*."
And I, I want to scream, *am only 41!*
How can this be happening to me?
Why can this man not look me in the eye?
Because he might find written there
A reflection of his own mortality?
The sky is falling!
I scramble from one waiting room to another,
Surrounded and unable to escape.
The old, the feeble-hearted, swap wretched tales of horror,
Celebrating cancer's evil march across their souls.
Voices of doom, one louder than the other,
Crying out, railing in a howl of discontent.

Underneath the radiologist's camera,
I stammer
Something about the Playboy centerfold
Being out of the question now.
Wrenched into a pretzeled twist, I try to deny the pinch of pain
As the wicked whir of X-rays bites into my breast,
What's left of it.
I say five "Hail Marys" and the camera is reset.

I was a redhead and it defined me.
In the hateful, horrid wig shop, with bodies inviolate,
Smug saleswomen coo, "Smile! Your picture for our records."
No wigs *my* color, best they can do is blonde.
Red has to be ordered, takes a couple of weeks.

Time, time, time. Never enough.
Adriamycin gallops through my veins.
I leave the wig shop a blonde.
Dolly Parton without the principal parts!

Mouth pierced with ulcers, head pounding, throat raw,
Temperature rises.
Back to the hospital in strictest isolation.
No fresh fruits or vegetables, no flowers.
My child visits swathed in a surgical mask.
My priest is told to wash his hands.
I sneer to the oncologist that I will come as a laboratory rat for Halloween.

"The sky is falling!" I scream to my husband,
Scared beyond all imagining.
"The sky *has* fallen," he whispers, holding onto me and my sanity
As I slip
Over the edge.

The white count rebounds,
More chemo.
Ignominious despair of parking under the sign
"Cancer Patients Only."
Technicians squirm.
Who will draw the woman with
The hidden, impenetrable veins?
Adriamycin, cold and caustic, etches its way
Like acid—like Drano—up my left arm.
("Your good arm, the one on the other side.")
Chatty nurses avoid my eyes,
Their children, after all, are older still than mine.

Hiding from myself.
Draping washcloths over the faucet
Lest I catch my bald reflection.
Cowering on the floor,

Putting on the hideous white turban or the wig,
Where I was sure not to see myself in the mirror.
Ah, the gut-wrenching fear of a coward and her wicked vanity.

Fevered writhing,
Racing through the night again to the ER,
Past the innocent twinkle of Christmas lights—
In happy, unknowing homes.
The usual chest X-ray.
If I arrived with a broken leg,
We would still need that chest X-ray first.
The interminable wait for the blood test.
People pop in and out.
Some know me, my veins,
Scurry away on some imagined errand.
Others, fools entrapped, try—
Call for back up.
The long wait for the blood count.
So few white cells, how can counting take so long?

Tucked away in my lonely room,
Scarlet blood drips into parched veins,
AIDS from a transfusion? Least of my worries.
My only company the Catholic channel on TV.
Maybe there are no atheists in foxholes,
But there aren't any on the cancer wards, either!
Days dribble by. White count stays flat.
Carolers fill the halls.
I did that as a child.
Sing Christmas carols to old people, in hospitals,
Waiting to die.
Strains of "Silent Night" float through my closed door.
The loneliest sound I've ever heard,
Before or since.
TV nuns watch over me through another harrowing night.

The healing hand of my blessed priest did
What medicines and doctors could not.
As Christ raised Lazarus, so Father raised my white count!
Home for Christmas.

Years pass.
God grants me the blessing of seeing my child grow up.
I remember a very sixties banner from my college dorm room—
"Tomorrow is the first day of the rest of your life."
Now I grasp its meaning.
Now I understand I have been blessed.
Yes, breast cancer was a blessing.
I learned what is important.
And what is not.
I have been blessed with the delicious freedom of celebrating my
life
One day at a time.

A freelance writer and novelist, Marie Fowler reviews the visual arts in the Philadelphia Main Line suburbs and has volunteered as a guide in museums in San Francisco, Singapore, Bangkok and Philadelphia.

Afterword
Breast Reconstruction
Malcolm Z. Roth, M.D

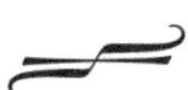

Of all of the different types of plastic surgery I perform, I receive the greatest professional and personal rewards from breast reconstruction. I am grateful for the opportunity to help restore and, in many cases, improve a patient's body image and self-esteem in circumstances where the patient has been told not only that she has cancer, but that she will lose one or both of her breasts in the course of treating the disease. In my experience, just knowing that reconstruction is possible can have a profoundly positive effect on a patient's treatment and recovery.

Federal law now requires that if a woman's health insurance provides coverage for mastectomy in the event of cancer, it must also cover reconstruction. In fact, all of the stages of reconstruction, which are discussed below, must by law be covered by insurance. Therefore, any discussion of cancer treatment options that involve the prospect of losing a breast should include a discussion about the option of breast reconstruction.

Although most breast surgeons are very familiar with breast reconstruction, the many different types of reconstruction now available warrant a consultation with a *board certified plastic sur-*

geon who has received additional training in reconstructive surgery, has been certified by the American Board of Plastic Surgery and is a member of the American Society of Plastic Surgeons. You can easily check the certification of any plastic surgeon by calling the American Society of Plastic Surgeons at 1-888-4PLASTIC or you can check the surgeon's certification online at www.plastic-surgery.org. For those who decide to proceed with reconstruction, the plastic surgeon becomes a vital part of the breast cancer team. In fact, because the reconstruction procedure is performed in several stages, the plastic surgeon is often the physician with whom the patient has the most contact during the course of her treatment.

The goal of breast reconstruction is to create a soft, natural looking, reconstructed breast. Over the past forty-five years, the medical community has made great progress towards achieving this goal. *Breast implants* first began to be used for breast reconstruction in the early 1970's and both *saline* (physiologic saltwater filled) and *silicone gel-filled* breast implants have been in use in breast reconstruction for many years. In 1992, the United States Food and Drug Administration removed silicone gel-filled implants from the market, except for women who chose to be part of an ongoing implant study, due to concerns raised about potential health risks. In 2006, after careful consideration of the scientific evidence and public testimony regarding the risks posed by the then-available silicone implants, the F.D.A. recommended that they be made freely available to all women. A tremendous amount of useful information about implants can be found at www.breast-implantsafety.org, or by calling the American Society of Plastic Surgeons.

If a patient decides to have reconstruction, she will meet with the plastic surgeon for an initial consultation, at which time the surgeon will take the patient's medical history and perform a physical examination. Afterwards, the surgical options will be discussed and the pros and cons of an *immediate* or *delayed reconstruction* will be outlined. In most instances, reconstruction can begin at the time of the *mastectomy*, the removal of the breast, and this procedure is known as immediate reconstruction. Occasionally and for several reasons the procedure is delayed and performed at a later time. Immediate reconstruction generally allows women to return to work and their normal social activities sooner than does delayed reconstruction. The best option for each woman is arrived at only after careful consideration of her anatomy, medical condition, personal preferences and the plastic surgeon's knowledge and experience.

Reconstruction using an implant is most often performed in stages. During the first stage, the surgeon will place a *tissue expander*, an inflatable implant, under the skin and *pectoralis major* (chest) muscle. Over the next several weeks, the plastic surgeon fills the tissue expander with salt water (*saline*) until the skin has stretched far enough to receive the permanent implant. During the second stage, which may be performed as an *outpatient procedure*, with no hospital stay needed, the expander is removed and a permanent saline or silicone gel-filled implant is inserted in its place. Occasionally, a tissue expander that can be left permanently in place is used in the first stage. If a *skin sparing mastectomy* has been performed, a procedure to remove a small amount of skin to prevent the further spread of cancer but leaving enough tissue to accommodate an implant, placement of a permanent implant is sometimes possible at the first stage, without the need for expansion. Reconstruction of the nipple and the *areola*, the dark skin surrounding the nipple, is the final stage to reconstruction of the breast.

For some women, an implant is not used. Instead, reconstruction of the breast mound is performed using the woman's own tissue, known as a *flap*, a procedure that can usually be performed at the time of the mastectomy. With this procedure, skin, fat and a muscle, the blood supply for which is left intact, are transferred from the patient's back or abdomen under the skin to the chest. If muscle from the abdomen is used, an added benefit can be an improved abdominal contour as unwanted, overhanging fat and skin can be removed and used to reconstruct the breast. On occasion, the flap might be transferred to the chest using *microsurgery*, attaching the blood vessels of the muscle and its overlying fat and skin to blood vessels under the arm or near the sternum with the assistance of a microscope or high-powered magnification glasses. Again, a full discussion of the procedure that is best for the patient must be had prior to surgery.

After the breast mound has been reconstructed, the other breast is often lifted, reduced or augmented in order to achieve better symmetry with the reconstructed breast. This is sometimes done in combination with nipple and areola reconstruction or breast implant exchange.

There are certainly risks associated with breast reconstruction, as there are with any operation. Portions of the flap might not survive, and rarely, the entire flap can be lost. Implants can become firm due to scar tissue that forms around the implant, and saline and silicone implants can leak, requiring replacement. The potential risks should be discussed with the plastic surgeon before surgery. Reconstruction with flaps usually requires a longer stay in the hospital, but the second stage procedure to exchange an expander for a permanent implant is avoided. However, for some women, a second stage procedure to modify the flap to create better shape is sometimes performed. In either case, the second stage may be performed as an outpatient procedure, and might only require local anesthesia. Recovery is generally easier for the later stages of reconstruction, with less need for pain medication.

Regardless of the type of reconstruction performed, it is important to maintain close follow-up with your plastic surgeon. Regular appointments will help assure that the recovery goes smoothly. An open discussion about resuming physical activities will minimize the chance of post-operative problems and maximize the possibility of a successful reconstruction and the happiness of the patient.

Dr. Malcolm Z. Roth has served as the Director of the Division of Plastic Surgery of Maimonides Medical Center located in New York City since 2005 after seventeen years at The Brookdale University Hospital and Medical Center, where he served as the Director of Plastic Surgery and Hand Surgery.

A graduate of the University of Pennsylvania and the medical school at New York Medical College, he trained in General Surgery at Beth Israel Medical Center in New York and completed plastic surgery training at The New York Hospital-Cornell University Medical Center. He also completed a fellowship in hand surgery at The Hospital for Special Surgery.

Dr. Roth is a past President of the New York Society for Surgery of the Hand and is a past Chair of the Government Affairs Council of the American Society of Plastic Surgeons. He is a member of the Board of Directors the American Society of Plastic Surgeons and has served on The American Society for Aesthetic Plastic Surgery Breast Implant Task Force.

Afterword
Breast Cancer: A Look Forward
Ellen Chuang, M.D.

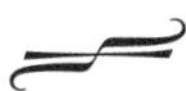

As we enter the 21st century, breast cancer continues to be the most common cancer diagnosed and the second leading cause of cancer deaths in women. Each year in the United States about 170,000 new cases of invasive breast cancer are diagnosed and 40,000 women will die of breast cancer. Yet breast cancer is one of the oldest known diseases, having first been written about in Egypt in 1600 BC. For centuries, there was no treatment for this dreaded disease. It was not until early in the 20th century, with the development of the surgical technique known as the *radical mastectomy*, pioneered by Dr. William S. Halsted of Johns Hopkins College of Medicine, together with the discovery of antibiotics and advances in anesthesia, that surgeons were able to successfully operate on women with breast cancer, giving women the first hope for a cure.

In the course of his experiences, Dr. Halsted noted that women who presented with small tumors in the breast that had not metastasized, or spread to the lymph nodes at the time of surgery, had a better prognosis for survival than did women who presented with large tumors or lymph node metastasis. These observations formed the basis for the first breast cancer staging system and led to the recognition of the need for early detection and of the need for *systemic* treatment, in addition to surgery, to help prevent the recurrence of the disease.

Building on these early observations, medical science in the 20th century laid the foundation for the modern treatment of breast cancer with the development of less radical surgical techniques, including *lumpectomy*, a procedure used to conserve as much of the breast as possible, *screening mammography*, developed in the 1970's for early tumor detection, and *adjuvant hormonal therapy* and *chemotherapy*, developed in the 1980's to slow the growth and spread of cancer tumors and prevent their recurrence. The steady increase in breast cancer survival rates since the 1990's attests to the remarkable success of these programs.

Where do we go from here? What does the future hold? In the past two decades there has been an explosion of knowledge in the fields of breast cancer biology, genetics, and epidemiology. These advances hold great promise, and are just now being translated into better treatments for our patients. The following describes only some of the breakthroughs that are creating new paradigms for the treatment and prevention of breast cancer in the 21st century.

Understanding Cancer Cell Growth

Together with ever more refined surgical and early detection techniques, it is our understanding of what drives breast cancer cells to grow that will soon radically alter the landscape of breast cancer treatment. When scientists learned to manipulate DNA, to cut and paste individual human genes, it became possible for the first time to study the genetic blueprint of every human cell. From this work, scientists discovered that cancer arises when *mutations*, or aberrations, occur in normal genes. Many of these aberrations occur in genes that regulate cell growth and are the agents responsible for turning a normal breast cell into a cancerous one which grows unchecked. One such mutation leading to cancer cell growth affects the protein found in the body known as *Her2/neu.* Her2/neu is a member of a family of proteins called the *epidermal growth factor receptors.* It is found at high levels on the surface of cancer cells in about 20% of women with breast cancer. Scientists observed that when Her2/neu was present, the cancer tended to be more aggressive. Scientists designed a *monoclonal antibody* named trastuzumab (Herceptin®) that could block the growth-inducing properties of Her2/neu. This was the first example of a "designer drug" or *targeted therapy* that is used only when cancer cells express the "target" (in this case, Her2/neu). Although Her2/neu was first described in the 1980's, it was not until 2005 that Herceptin® began to be used in the adjuvant setting (that is, treatment after surgery to prevent recurrence) and only after clinical trials held in the U.S. and Europe showed that there was a dramatic reduction of breast cancer recurrences in women who were treated with Herceptin® after surgery.

Since the discovery of Her2/neu, many more targets have been identified and drugs to block these targets are rapidly being developed. New biologic therapies available or soon to be available for the treatment of breast cancer include lapatinib (Tykerb®), which has been shown to be effective in patients whose tumors no longer respond to Herceptin®, and bevacizumab (Avastin®), an *antiangiogenesis* drug which limits tumor growth by stopping the formation of tumor-related blood vessels that provide critical nutrients to the tumor.

The Discovery of the BRCA Genes

In 1990, scientists performed DNA studies on large, extended families in which many members were affected by breast cancer and in which breast cancer seemed to be passed down from generation to generation. Through this work scientists identified the first gene to be associated with breast cancer, now known as "breast cancer 1" or *BRCA1*. However, since many families who had inherited forms of breast cancer did not have a mutation in the BRCA1 gene, studies continued and, in 1994, scientists discovered another gene (similar to BRCA1), and named it *BRCA2*. Both BRCA1 and BRCA2 are *tumor suppressor* genes that usually act to control cell growth and cell death. Mutations in these genes which prevent their ability to function are now routinely tested for in breast cancer patients who have a family history of breast cancer or ovarian cancer, develop breast cancer at an early age, or have breast cancers in both breasts. It is estimated that 10,000 women each year are diagnosed with BRCA1 or BRCA2-related tumors. If a mutation is found, a woman (and, importantly, her relatives) can be counseled about the risk of a recurrence of breast cancer or of ovarian cancer, and what can be done to monitor for these cancers or to prevent them altogether. If women carrying the BRCA mutations can be identified early, they can take appropriate action. Such actions include *prophylactic mastectomy*, breast removal before the onset of cancer, which is 95% effective in preventing breast cancer, or *prophylactic oopherectomy*, the removal of the ovaries, which not only prevents ovarian cancer but also reduces the risk of breast cancer by 50% when performed in premenopausal BRCA mutation carriers. Alternatively, women with the BRCA mutation may choose to undergo intensive screening procedures, such as with *breast MRI*, so that if a cancer does develop, it will be detected early and in the most treatable stages.

A strong family history of breast cancer remains one of the best indicators of increased breast cancer risk in a woman. However, less than half of women who have a familial form of breast cancer will test positive for one of the known BRCA 1 or 2 gene mutations. Geneticists are now working hard to find a "BRCA3" gene to account for these cases, but have not been successful to date. It may not exist. Instead, scientists are discovering mutations in genes that cause a more modest increase in breast cancer risk. Currently, the most promising of these candidates include genes known as CHEK1, ATM, and RAD 50. While BRCA 1 or BRCA2 mutations lead to a 10-fold increase in risk of developing breast cancer, mutations in these other genes lead to a 2-fold increase in risk. At present, clinical testing for only the CHEK2 mutation is available. Patients who carry mutations in these genes may be candidates for more intensive pharmacological or lifestyle interventions and more intensive screening to decrease their risk.

Modifying the Modern Lifestyle

In 1713, an Italian physician observed that breast cancer disproportionately affected nuns, and wondered if it was their celibate lifestyle that predisposed them to the disease. We now know that the reason nuns are more likely to develop breast cancer is because women who have never been pregnant are at higher risk for the disease. We also know that, in addition to the number of pregnancies, age at menarche and age at first birth also influence breast cancer risk. Unfortunately, risk factors such as family history and reproductive history either cannot be modified (family history), or cannot be modified in practical terms (reproductive history). However, there are several risk factors for breast cancer that *can* be modified. They include obesity, sedentary lifestyle, alcohol use, and the use of *exogenous* hormones.

A striking example of how breast cancer incidence can be reduced in a population is illustrated by the story of *hormone replacement therapy* (HRT) in postmenopausal women. Millions of women in the 1990's were treated with HRT for menopausal symptoms. In 2002, when results from the Women's Health Initiative study showed that women who used estrogen and progestin were more likely to experience a cardiac event as well as breast cancer, large numbers of women stopped taking HRT. In 2003, the incidence of breast cancer decreased for the first time. This decrease has been attributed primarily to the decrease in HRT use by postmenopausal women.

In the United States, it is estimated that obesity is responsible for nearly 8% of all breast cancers, and 11% of all breast cancers can be attributable to lack of physical activity. Taken together, nearly 20% of all breast cancers could be prevented if obesity was eliminated and if women could be persuaded to engage in at least moderate levels of exercise. Clearly, obesity and the lack of exercise are serious health problems which, if successfully tackled in the future, would not only lead to a reduction in breast cancer incidence but also a reduction in the incidence of diabetes, cardiovascular disease, and hypertension. This is a big challenge, but as the medical community and the government recognize the magnitude of the obesity epidemic, more financial resources will surely be employed in the future to find innovative ways to address this problem.

Breast Cancer Is Not Just One Disease: Individualizing Breast Cancer Treatment

If there is one attainable goal for the 21st century, it is that we will be able to individualize adjuvant treatment for the breast cancer patient. Today, chemotherapy drugs are chosen for use based upon testing done in large clinical trials: a few drugs are tested on large populations of women with breast cancer and if a drug is found to improve the average outcome of the study population, it is approved by the FDA for use. In these large clinical trials, some patients gain quite a bit of benefit from the treatment, while others do not benefit at all. The goal of the near future will be to tease out of the population those patients who will not benefit from the drug so that other drugs may be tested and developed for this specific group. A step in the right direction has been made through the use of recently developed *gene profiling techniques*. By using sophisticated statistical analyses, scientists have been able to break down breast cancer into about five or six subtypes, based upon which genes are turned on and turned off compared with normal, noncancerous breast cells. These classifications can be important for two reasons. First, scientists can work to discover drugs to specifically target and reverse these aberrant patterns. Second, at the population level, by recognizing that breast cancer is many diseases and that certain drugs may be effective for one type of breast cancer but not for another, clinicians will be able to better design their studies to test new therapies on populations of women with the same type of breast cancer. This will increase the likelihood that effective treatments for that group will not be missed.

Pharmacogenomics

Pharmacogenomics is the study of the differences in the genetic makeup of people that determine how effective a drug will be and what type of side effects a drug may cause in particular people. One of the best examples of how pharmacogenomics is likely to influence breast cancer treatment is illustrated by recent studies on a gene known as CYP2D6. CYP2D6 is an enzyme which converts tamoxifen, a drug widely used to slow or stop the growth of breast cancer cells, into one of its active forms, allowing it to work in the body. About 10% of the population in the United States has a version of the CYP2D6 gene that does not perform this function very well. For these patients, tamoxifen will not be as effective as it will be for patients who have the more common version of CYP2D6, and therefore it might not be the best choice of therapy for them. Doctors are still trying to determine how best to use this information. CYP2D6 gene variants are being tested at the Mayo Clinic in postmenopausal women who can choose between tamoxifen treatment and other hormonal therapies. This test is not for premenopausal women, for which tamoxifen is the *only* choice for hormonal therapy.

Pharmacogenomics is also being used to identify individuals who may benefit more from one chemotherapy drug over another. For instance, preliminary studies show that patients with many copies of a certain gene known as *topoisomerase II* gain the most benefit from adriamycin, a very common breast cancer drug. If this gene was present in low copy numbers, there is little advantage to using the drug. And, because adriamycin has unique side effects, it would be best to avoid its use in patients who would not be expected to benefit. To be able to choose which drug is most likely to benefit a patient *before* it is used has obvious advantages: rather than trying all keys to find the right one that fits the lock, we will have the technology to choose the right key from the very start. We expect many more breakthroughs from pharmacogenomics in the not too distant future.

This is an exciting time for breast cancer researchers and doctors. For patients who have breast cancer, there is the promise of more effective and more individualized treatments on the horizon. More recurrences will be prevented, and more lives saved. One of the greatest challenges for the future will be to find better treatments for patients whose cancers have *metastasized*, or spread outside the breast. During the 1990's, for the first time in the history of breast cancer treatment, drugs were found which extended the lives of women with metastatic cancer. Today, the topic of breast cancer metastases is one of the most intensely studied by scientists. With continued progress, the treatment of metastastic breast cancer like a chronic illness may be a realistic goal for patients and the medical community alike.

Ellen Chuang is an Assistant Professor of Clinical Medicine at the Weill Cornell Medical College in New York City. An oncologist and clinical researcher, she is a past recipient of a Clinical Investigator Award from the National Institutes of Health, and a Junior Faculty Award from the American Society of Hematology.

Resources

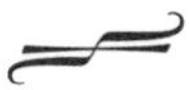

On the following pages you will find information on some of the foremost organizations in the country focused on breast cancer research, treatment and support. All of these and many, many more may be found within the Resources & Links section of The Healing Project's website at www.thehealingproject.org.

African-American Organizations

African American Women in Touch

574-647-1000
Memorial Hospital & Health System
615 N. Michigan St.
South Bend, IN 46601
http://www.qualityoflife.org

African American Women in Touch operates out of the Memorial Hospital & Health System in South Bend, Indiana. The organization educates African-American women about breast cancer, provides information on early detection, and offers free mammograms to women who cannot afford them. It also provides a network of support through its monthly meetings and annual health care symposium. African American Women in Touch provides women facing breast cancer with transportation to treatment, wigs and free prostheses.

Breast Cancer Resource Committee
202-463-8040
2005 Belmont St., NW
Washington, DC 20009
http://www.bcresource.org

The Breast Cancer Resource Committee is dedicated to reducing breast cancer incidence and mortality among African-American women. The organization advocates for mammography screening for African-American women aged 35 and older, emphasizes the importance of early detection, organizes support groups and offers peer counseling. The BCRC also educates African-American women about breast cancer through outreach initiatives such as Rise-Sister-Rise, which provides counseling and support services for women with breast cancer.

Living Beyond Breast Cancer
888-753-5222
10 East Athens Ave., Suite 204
Ardmore, PA 19003
http://www.lbbc.org

Living Beyond Breast Cancer offers educational programs and services to women and families affected by breast cancer. Its programs include a toll-free Survivors' Helpline (888-753-5222), a free quarterly newsletter, publications for African-American and Latina women, and networking programs for young survivors and women of color.

Sisters Network Inc.
713-781-0255
8787 Woodway Dr., Suite 4206
Houston, TX 77063
http://www.sistersnetwork.org

Sisters Network increases awareness about the impact breast cancer has on the African-American community. The organization provides African-American women with educational materials about breast cancer risk, symptoms and treatment. Sisters Network maintains support-group chapters in about two dozen states.

Asian-American Organizations

National Asian Women's Health Organization

415-773-2838
1 Embarcadero Center, Suite 500
San Francisco, CA 94111
http://www.nawho.org

The National Asian Women's Health Organization (NAWHO) aims to raise awareness about the health needs of Asian-American women. The organization's mission covers a wide range of health issues, including breast and cervical cancer. It created the Asian American Women's Breast and Cervical Cancer Project as a way to address the needs of Asian-American women living with breast and cervical cancers. The Project provides a list of Asian-language informational resources.

Jewish Organizations

JPAC Jewish Association for Services for the Aged (JASA)

212-273-5262 and 718-934-7718
132 West 31st St.
New York, NY 10001
http://www.jpac.org

Provides mammogram screenings at its senior centers.

Jewish Board of Family and Children's Services (JBFCS)

212-582-9100 and 888-523-2769
120 West 57th St.
New York, NY 10019
http://www.jbfcs.org

New York Jewish Healing Center of JBFCS provides support groups for women with breast and ovarian cancer and provides breast health education.

Sharsheret
866-474-2774
P.O. Box 3245
Teaneck, NJ 07666
http://www.sharsheret.org

Sharsheret is a national organization of cancer survivors that provides culturally sensitive support and information to Jewish women facing breast cancer. Sharsheret also offers specialized information for the friends and families of breast cancer patients and for women who have a high risk of developing the disease.

Latino Organizations

Nueva Vida, Inc.
202-223-9100
2000 P St., NW, Suite 740
Washington, DC 20036
http://www.nueva-vida.org

Nueva Vida is made up of Latina breast cancer survivors and Latino healthcare professionals who are committed to providing culturally sensitive support services for Latinas living with cancer in the Washington metropolitan area. Nueva Vida offers support, education and resources in both Spanish and English.

Living Beyond Breast Cancer
888-753-5222
10 East Athens Ave., Suite 204
Ardmore, PA 19003
http://www.lbbc.org

Living Beyond Breast Cancer offers educational programs and services to women and families affected by breast cancer. Its programs include a toll-free Survivors' Helpline (888-753-5222), a free quarterly newsletter, publications for African-American and Latina women, and networking programs for young survivors and women of color.

Organizations for Senior Women

DOROT, Inc.

212-769-2850
171 West 85th St.
New York, NY 10024
http://www.dorotusa.org

Offers programs for sick and frail seniors over age 60 including those with breast cancer.

Living Beyond Breast Cancer

888-753-5222
10 East Athens Ave., Suite 204
Ardmore, PA 19003
http://www.lbbc.org

Living Beyond Breast Cancer offers educational programs and services to women and families affected by breast cancer. Its programs include a toll-free Survivors' Helpline (888-753-5222), a free quarterly newsletter, publications for African-American and Latina women, and networking programs for young survivors and women of color.

Younger Women and Breast Cancer

Young Survival Coalition

212-206-6610
155 Sixth Ave., 10th Floor
New York, NY 10013
http://www.youngsurvival.org

The Young Survival Coalition (YSC) is dedicated to the concerns and issues that are unique to young women with breast cancer. YSC has an online bulletin board where young survivors can communicate with each other and it publishes informational brochures and a quarterly newsletter. The organization also has affiliate branches that host meetings in 12 states. In addition to educational and support services for survivors, YSC works to educate community and government officials about the unique issues affecting young women diagnosed with breast cancer.

Information on Male Breast Cancer

People Living with Cancer

American Society of Clinical Oncology
703-519-2927 and 888-651-3038
1900 Duke St., Suite 200
Alexandria, VA 22314
http://www.plwc.org

PLWC provides timely, oncologist-approved information to help patients and families make informed healthcare decisions. All content is subject to a formal peer-review process by the PLWC Editorial Board, comprised of over 135 medical, surgical and radiation oncologists, oncology nurses, social workers and patient advocates. In addition, ASCO editorial staff reviews the content for easy readability. PLWC content is reviewed on an annual basis or as needed.

Inflammatory Breast Cancer

Inflammatory Breast Cancer Research Foundation

877-STOP-IBC
http://www.ibcresearch.org

The Inflammatory Breast Cancer Research Foundation educates people about inflammatory breast cancer (IBC). Its website offers three e-mail discussion lists, a newsletter, a listing of IBC clinical trials, and other educational materials.

Nationwide Organizations Devoted to Breast Cancer

National Cancer Institute

800-4-CANCER (800-422-6237)
NCI Public Inquiries Office
6116 Executive Blvd., Room 3036A
Bethesda, MD 20892-8322
http://www.cancer.gov

The National Cancer Institute (NCI) is a component of the National Institutes of Health (NIH), one of eight agencies that comprise the Public Health Service of the Department of Health and Human Services. The NCI, established under the National Cancer Institute Act of 1937, is the Federal Government's principal agency for cancer research and training. The NCI coordinates the National Cancer Program, which conducts and supports research, training, health information dissemination, and other programs on the cause, diagnosis, prevention and treatment of cancer, rehabilitation from cancer, and the continuing care of cancer patients and the families of cancer patients.

Mayo Clinic

Jacksonville, Florida
4500 San Pablo Road
Jacksonville, FL 32224
General Telephone: 904-953-2000
Appointments: 904-953-0853
Hearing Impaired: 904-953-2300
http://www.mayoclinic.com

Rochester, Minnesota
200 First St. SW
Rochester, MN 55905
General Telephone: 507-538-3270
Appointments: 507-538-3270
Hearing Impaired: 507-281-9786
http://www.mayoclinic.com

Phoenix/Scottsdale, Arizona
Mayo Clinic Hospital
5777 East Mayo Blvd.
Phoenix, AZ 85054
480-515-6296
http://www.mayoclinic.com

Mayo Clinic Arizona
13400 East Shea Blvd.
Scottsdale, AZ 85259
480-301-8000
http://www.mayoclinic.com

The Mayo Clinic is a not-for-profit medical practice dedicated to the diagnosis and treatment of virtually every type of complex illness. Its three main websites provide information and services from the world's first and largest integrated, not-for-profit group medical practice. Manage your health with information and tools that reflect the expertise of Mayo's 2,500 physicians and scientists, learn how to access medical services and learn about Mayo's medical research and education offerings.

Susan G. Komen Breast Cancer Foundation
800-I'M AWARE (800-462-9273)
5005 LBJ Freeway, Suite 250
Dallas, TX 75244
http://www.komen.org

The Susan G. Komen Breast Cancer Foundation funds research grants and supports breast cancer education, screening and treatment projects in communities around the world through an extensive network of United States and international affiliates. The Foundation also provides information about breast health and breast cancer, treatment options and community support groups through a national toll-free helpline (800-I'M AWARE or 800-462-9273) and distributes a variety of educational materials to those affected by breast cancer.

National Alliance of Breast Cancer Organizations (NABCO)
9 East 37th St., 10th Floor
New York, NY 10016
http://www.nabco.org

A resource clearinghouse, it provides general information about breast cancer and phone numbers for more than 300 cancer support groups throughout the country and advocates for legislative concerns of breast cancer patients and survivors.

National Advocacy Programs

National Breast Cancer Coalition
800-622-2838
1101 17th St., NW, Suite 1300
Washington, DC 20036
http://www.natlbcc.org

The National Breast Cancer Coalition (NBCC) aims to eradicate breast cancer by focusing government, research institutions and consumer advocates on breast cancer. The coalition informs, trains and directs patients and others in effective advocacy efforts. NBCC's goals include promoting breast cancer research; improving access to high-quality breast cancer screening, diagnosis, treatment and care; and increasing the involvement and influence of breast cancer survivors and activists in the decision-making processes that impact the disease. The NBCC website provides a list of fact sheets, analyses and position papers related to breast cancer.

Breast Cancer Information

Breast Cancer Action

877-2STOPBC (877-278-6722)
55 New Montgomery St., Suite 323
San Francisco, CA 94105
http://www.bcaction.org

Breast Cancer Action (BCA) is a grassroots organization of breast cancer survivors and their supporters that educates people about breast cancer issues. The group publishes a bimonthly newsletter about breast cancer research and advocacy and its website has downloadable flyers and fact sheets on breast cancer issues. BCA also provides a booklet for newly diagnosed breast cancer patients.

The Breast Cancer Fund

415-346-8223
1388 Sutter St., Suite 400
San Francisco, CA 94109
http://www.breastcancerfund.org

The Breast Cancer Fund works to identify environmental and other preventable contributors to breast cancer and it advocates for their elimination. The fund, which also educates the public about cancer prevention, produces a quarterly newsletter, monthly e-newsletter and fact sheets, which are all available on its website. The organization also publishes informational brochures for the Latina community.

Breast Cancer Survivor Organizations

The National Coalition for Cancer Survivorship

301-650-9127

1010 Wayne Ave.
Suite 770
Silver Spring, MD 20910
http://www.canceradvocacy.org

Advocates on behalf of cancer patients and survivors.

Breast Cancer Research and Awareness

The Breast Cancer Research Foundation
866-FIND A CURE (866-346-3228)
60 East 56th St., Eighth Floor
New York, NY 10022
http://www.bcrfcure.org

The Breast Cancer Research Foundation is dedicated to preventing and curing breast cancer by raising funds for innovative research and increasing awareness of good breast health. The foundation has information on its website about how to find a clinical trial and it provides support resources for people living with breast cancer, including a special section of its website dedicated to men with breast cancer.

Information on Breast Cancer Treatment

Breast Cancer.org
111 Forrest Ave., #1R
Narberth, PA 19072
http://www.breastcancer.org

Breastcancer.org can help you understand your cancer stage and appropriate options, so you and your doctors can arrive at the best treatment plan for you.

Cancer.gov
National Cancer Institute
800-4-CANCER (800-422-6237)

NCI Public Inquiries Office
6116 Executive Blvd., Room 3036A
Bethesda, MD 20892-8322
http://www.cancer.gov

Treatment information from NCI on male and female breast cancer.

MD Anderson
877-MDA-6789
University of Texas M.D. Anderson Cancer Center
1515 Holcombe Blvd.
Houston, TX 77030
http://www.mdanderson.org

A comprehensive resource for breast cancer publications and information on treatment.

Information on Caregiving

National Family Caregivers Association
800-896-3650
10400 Connecticut Ave., Suite 500
Kensington, MD 20895-3944
http://www.nfcacares.org

Educates, supports, empowers and speaks up for the more than 50 million Americans who care for loved ones with a chronic illness or disability or the frailties of old age. NFCA reaches across the boundaries of diagnoses, relationships and life stages to address the common needs and concerns of all family caregivers.

Local Support and Advocacy Organizations

California
Between Women
760-351-1774
P.O. Box 1225

Brawley, CA 92227
http://www.betweenwomen.net

Between Women is the only advocacy, educational and support organization in California's Imperial Valley devoted exclusively to breast health. It provides support services for local women undergoing treatment for breast cancer and is dedicated to promoting awareness and education about the disease throughout the community. Members also advocate with legislators for better laws for breast cancer patients.

Massachusetts

Lotsa Helping Hands
978-835-6080
365 Boston Post Road, Suite 157
Sudbury, MA 01776
http://www.lotsahelpinghands.com

Provides online an easy-to-use, private group calendar specifically designed for organizing helpers, where everyone can pitch in with meals delivery, rides, and other tasks necessary for life to run smoothly during a crisis.

New York

The Educational Alliance
212-780-2300
197 East Broadway
New York, NY 10002
http://www.edalliance.org

Dedicated to serving those most in need, especially those who are going through times of great challenge, stress or trauma.

The Libby Ross Foundation
212-658-9031
351 East 84th St., Suite 25E
New York, NY 10028
http://www.thelibbyrossfoundation.com

Provides gift bags distributed by trained volunteers to women recently diagnosed with breast cancer. The program is currently offered at New York Presbyterian Hospital and The Comprehensive Breast Center at St. Luke's Roosevelt Hospital; offers free weekly classes, quarterly workshops and semiannual weekend retreats for survivors of breast cancer and other women's cancers. The Foundation has partnered with OM yoga center in New York to offer breast cancer survivors an opportunity to bond with other women who have had or who are currently being treated for the disease.

1 in 9: The Long Island Breast Cancer Action Coalition
516-374-3190
CC/Nassau County Medical Center
2201 Hempstead Turnpike
East Meadow, NY 11554
http://www.1in9.org

An organization that promotes breast cancer awareness through education, outreach, advocacy and research support to find the causes and cures for breast cancer.

SHARE: Self-help for Women with Breast or Ovarian Cancer
866-891-2392
1501 Broadway, Suite 704A
New York, NY 10036
http://www.sharecancersupport.org

SHARE offers support to women with breast or ovarian cancer in the New York metropolitan area. Cancer survivors lead SHARE's support groups and staff its hotlines. There are separate hotlines for breast and ovarian Latina patients; programs for families and friends affected by breast and ovarian cancer; and workshops for patients in yoga, qigong, Chinese medicine and holistic health. SHARE offers educational programs on topics such as lymphedema, clinical trials, bone health, hormonal treatments, access to medical care and advocacy.

Ohio

Pink Ribbon Girls
513-207-7975
P.O. Box 33011
Cincinnati, OH 45233
http://www.pinkribbongirls.org

859-230-1175
P.O. Box 11995
Lexington, KY 40579

A nonprofit organization committed to helping young women diagnosed with breast cancer by creating an online support network of survivors via a national searchable database of survivors, private message boards, and electronic newsletters.

Pennsylvania

Linda Creed Breast Cancer Foundation
877-99-CREED (877-992-7333)
1601 Walnut St., Suite 1418
Philadelphia, PA 19102-2909
http://www.lindacreed.org

The Linda Creed Breast Cancer Foundation offers financial assistance to women in the Philadelphia region receiving breast cancer treatment. The Foundation also provides women and their families with informational materials and access to detection and treatment resources.

Texas

The Rose
The ROSE Diagnostic Center
The Rose Medical Plaza
12700 North Featherwood
Suite 260
Houston, TX 77034
281-484-4708

The ROSE Joan Gordon Center
3400 Bissonnet
Suite 185
Houston, TX 77005
713-668-2996
http://www.the-rose.org

Founded in 1986, the mission of The Rose is to reduce deaths from breast cancer by providing screening, diagnosis and access to treatment to women regardless of their ability to pay.

Explaining Cancer to Children

Hurricane Voices
866-667-3300
1340 Centre St., Suite 208
Newton, MA 02459
http://www.hurricanevoices.org

Hurricane Voices is a breast cancer foundation that works to educate men and women about the reality of breast cancer through advertising campaigns and educational materials. The foundation publishes news articles about breast cancer on its website as well as in a triannual newsletter. Hurricane Voices also offers a listing of books that parents can use to explain cancer to their children.

Free or Affordable Breast Cancer Screening

CDC National Breast and Cervical Cancer Early Detection Program
800-311-3435
404-639-3534 (public inquiries) 404-639-3311 (switchboard)
1600 Clifton Road
Atlanta, GA 30333
http://www.cdc.gov

Through this program, the Center for Disease Control and Prevention (CDC) provides low-income, uninsured and underserved women access to timely, high-quality screening and diagnostic services to detect breast and cervical cancer at the earliest stages.

Travel Assistance

Corporate Angel Network

866-328-1313
Westchester County Airport
1 Loop Road
White Plains, NY 10604-1215
http://www.corpangelnetwork.org

The only charitable organization in the U.S. whose sole mission is to ease the emotional stress, physical discomfort and financial burden of travel for cancer patients by arranging free flights to treatment centers, using the empty seats on corporate aircraft flying on routine business.

Wigs or Prostheses

Y-ME—Wig and Prosthesis Bank

312-986-8338
Helplines: 800-221-2141 (English) and 800-986-9505 (Spanish)
212 W. Van Buren St., Suite 1000
Chicago, IL 60607-3903
http://www.y-me.org

Y-ME provides wigs and prostheses free of charge for women with limited resources.

Hospice Care

Hospice Foundation of America

680-854-3402
http://www.hospicefoundation.org

Hospice Foundation of America provides leadership in the development and application of hospice and its philosophy of care with the goal of enhancing the American healthcare system and the role of hospice within it.

National Hospice and Palliative Care Organization
703-837-1500
Helpline: 800-658-8898
Espanol: 877-658-8896
1700 Diagonal Road, #625
Alexandria, VA 22314
http://www.nhpco.org

An extensive listing of resources for people with all types of cancer.

Send Us Your Story

Do you have a story to tell? LaChance Publishing and The Healing Project publish four books a year of stories written by people like you. Have you or those you know been touched by life-threatening illness or chronic disease? Your story can give comfort, courage and strength to others who are going through what you have already faced.

Your story should be no less than 500 words and no more than 2,000 words. You can write about yourself or someone you know. Your story must inform, inspire or teach others. Tell the story of how you or someone you know faced adversity; what you learned that would be important for others to know; how dealing with the disease strengthened or clarified your relationships or inspired positive changes in your life.

The easiest way to submit your story is to visit The Healing Project website at www.thehealingproject.com or the LaChance Publishing website at www.lachancepublishing.com. There you will find guidelines for submitting your story online, or you may write to us at submissions@lachancepublishing.com. We look forward to reading your story!

For the duration of the printing and circulation of this book, for every book that is sold by LaChance Publishing, LaChance will contribute 100% of the net proceeds to The Healing Project, Inc. The Healing Project can be reached at Five Laurel Road, South Salem, NY 10590. The Healing Project is dedicated to promoting the health and well-being of individuals suffering from life-threatening illnesses and chronic diseases and developing resources to enhance the quality of life of such individuals and assisting the family members and friends who care for them. The Healing Project is a nonprofit 501(c)(3) organization.